Atlas of Mitral Valve Repair

Atlas of Mitral Valve Repair

AUTHORS

EDWARD B. SAVAGE, MD

Associate Professor of Cardiovascular-Thoracic Surgery
Rush University
Chairman, Division of Cardiothoracic Surgery
John H. Stroger, Jr. Hospital of Cook County
Chicago, Illinois

STEVEN F. BOLLING, MD

Professor of Surgery
Section of Cardiac Surgery
Gayle Halperin Kahn Professor Integrative Medicine
University of Michigan
Ann Arbor, Michigan

. Lippincott Williams & Wilkins
a Wolters Kluwer business

Philadelphia · Baltimore · New York · London
Buenos Aires · Hong Kong · Sydney · Tokyo

Acquisitions Editor: Brian Brown
Managing Editor: Julia Seto
Project Manager: Alicia Jackson
Senior Manufacturing Manager: Benjamin Rivera
Associate Director of Marketing: Adam Glazer
Creative Director: Doug Smock
Cover Designer: Karen Quigley
Production Service: Nesbitt Graphics, Inc.
Printer: Quebecor World—Kingsport

© 2006 by LIPPINCOTT WILLIAMS & WILKINS
530 Walnut Street
Philadelphia, PA 19106 USA
LWW.com

Library of Congress Cataloging-in-Publication Data

Savage, Edward Bruce.
  Atlas of mitral valve repair / Edward B. Savage, Steven F. Bolling.
    p. ; cm.
  Includes index.
  ISBN–13: 978-0-7817-4692-2
  1. Mitral valve—Surgery—Atlases. I. Bolling, Steven. II. Title.
  [DNLM: 1. Heart Valve Diseases—surgery—Atlases. 2. Mitral
Valve—surgery—Atlases. 3. Cardiac Surgical Procedures—methods—Atlases.
WG 17 S263a 2006]
  RD598.S29 2006
  617.4'12—dc22   2005025874

Care has been taken to confirm the accuracy of the information presented and to describe generally accepted practices. However, the authors, editors, and publisher are not responsible for errors or omissions or for any consequences from application of the information in this book and make no warranty, expressed or implied, with respect to the currency, completeness, or accuracy of the contents of the publication. Application of the information in a particular situation remains the professional responsibility of the practitioner.

The authors, editors, and publisher have exerted every effort to ensure that drug selection and dosage set forth in this text are in accordance with current recommendations and practice at the time of publication. However, in view of ongoing research, changes in government regulations, and the constant flow of information relating to drug therapy and drug reactions, the reader is urged to check the package insert for each drug for any change in indications and dosage and for added warnings and precautions. This is particularly important when the recommended agent is a new or infrequently employed drug.

Some drugs and medical devices presented in the publication have Food and Drug Administration (FDA) clearance for limited use in restricted research settings. It is the responsibility of the health care provider to ascertain the FDA status of each drug or device planned for use in their clinical practice.

To purchase additional copies of this book, call our customer service department at (800) 638-3030 or fax orders to (301) 223-2320. International customers should call (301) 223-2300.

Visit Lippincott Williams & Wilkins on the Internet: at LWW.com. Lippincott Williams & Wilkins customer service representatives are available from 8:30 am to 6 pm, EST.

10 9 8 7 6 5 4 3

For their patience and support—Susan, Jennifer, Matthew
and Jonathan
Edward B. Savage, MD

Dedicated to my children, Michael and Kate
Steven F. Bolling, MD

Contents

Preface

Mitral valve repair was one of the first operations performed on the heart. In 1923 Elliot Cutler performed a successful valvotomy for mitral stenosis.[1] Though this was a destructive rather than a reconstructive procedure, it nevertheless is the first representation of the concept behind mitral valve repair—to use the patients own valvular tissue to create a functional, durable treatment for the affecting disease process. When valve prostheses were developed the surgeon's attention was temporarily diverted from repair. Prostheses were easier to place and required less ischemic time. However, the early enthusiasm for bioprostheses was tempered by their limited life span. Enthusiasm for mechanical prostheses was tempered by the requirement for anticoagulation. A few pioneers continued to develop and refine techniques and demonstrated that repair led to lower failure rates with a lower incidence of thromboembolism, hemorrhage, and infection. Despite this repair is probably underutilized by U.S. surgeons.[2]

This book was conceived to foster and promote the application of repair techniques in mitral surgery. Because busy surgeons do not have much spare time we aimed for brevity. The stated goal at the outset was not to recommend, but instead to review and assess the wide variety of techniques surgeons have applied over the years to treat different problems. The book is organized based on techniques that address problems with specific valve components, attempting to present a number of solutions for similar problems. Since static diagrams often do not transfer well to the operating room we have included six complete annotated videos to supplement the text. However, unlike many video presentations, we have broken these up into specific segments with references within the text. We have included certain images from the video in the text to emphasize key points. These can be identified by the film strip icon ▥ in the legend.

For surgeons who perform mitral repair we hope this will be a nice review and perhaps add some new techniques to your armamentarium. For those just beginning to learn we hope this provides a suitable roadmap for your journey.

Edward B. Savage M.D., St. Louis, MO
Steven F. Bolling M.D., Ann Arbor, MI

1. Cutler EC, Levine SA: Cardiotomy and valvulotomy for mitral stenosis. *Boston Med Surg J.* 1923; 188:1023.
2. Savage EB, Ferguson Jr. TB, DiSesa VJ: Use of Mitral Valve Repair: Analysis of Contemporary United States Experience Reported to the Society of Thoracic Surgeons National Cardiac Database. *Ann Thorac Surg.* 75:820-5, 2003.

Atlas of Mitral Valve Repair

The Natural History of Mitral Regurgitation

PHYSIOLOGY OF NORMAL VALVE FUNCTION

The function of the mitral valve is determined by atrial and ventricular volumes and pressure gradients, atrial and ventricular muscular contraction and relaxation, and the structural and functional integrity of the leaflets and chords. At the end of systole when the mitral valve is closed and the aortic valve is open, the ventricle begins to relax. The aortic valve quickly closes and the period of isovolumic relaxation begins. When the ventricular pressure falls below that of the atrium, the mitral valve opens and the rapid or early ventricular filling phase begins. More than two thirds of the eventual stroke volume enters the ventricle at this time (1). As the pressure gradient equalizes, the period of diastasis begins where there is little flow and the leaflets tend to move toward each other. With atrial contraction, the remainder of the stroke volume (generally less than 25% of the total stroke volume) is pushed into the ventricle to complete filling. After atrial contraction, the atrial pressure falls, this, along with the associated increase in ventricular pressure from systolic contraction, rapidly forces the valve into its closed position, entering the period of isovolumic ventricular contraction. Until the aortic valve opens, the back pressure on the mitral valve pushes it into the atrium. Continued contraction pulls the valve ring and valve towards the apex, reducing atrial pressure and promoting atrial filling. At the completion of ventricular systole the valve apparatus moves back towards the atrium and the process begins again. Each anatomical part of the valve contributes to this process, which is further detailed in Chapter 2.

REGURGITATION AS THE FINAL COMMON PATHWAY

Mitral regurgitation is the final common pathway of many disease processes. Damage to the valve leaflets or support structures leads to incompetence of the valve whether minor or major, which causes progression through ventricular dilatation, annular dilatation and impaired annular contraction, leaflet and chordal damage to increasing degrees of insufficiency, and progressive ventricular dysfunction. Chronic insufficiency leads to pulmonary hypertension (at first reversible then irreversible), associated right heart dilatation, tricuspid regurgitation, and eventually right heart failure. Whatever the etiology, most patients with severe mitral regurgitation have a contributing component of annular dilatation that must be corrected as part of the repair. One scenario in which annular dilatation may not be a component of the pathophysiology is acute ischemia-induced mitral insufficiency, though chronic ischemic insufficiency is generally associated with annular dilatation. This absence of annular dilatation in the acute setting makes successful repair less likely than in the chronic situation in which dilatation has occurred. Other scenarios in which annular dilatation may not be significant include endocarditis or chordal rupture with acute regurgitation and rheumatic disease in which the fibrotic disease process prevents annular enlargement.

The Development of Mitral Surgery

The understanding of mitral valve structure, function, and pathophysiology has evolved significantly over the past thirty years. The first reports of repair using an open approach on cardiopulmonary bypass were published in 1957 (2,3) with the first description of repair of incompetence caused by a ruptured chordae in 1960 (4). These predated the first successful mitral valve replacement reported in 1961 (5). The first mitral valve replacements required removal of all parts of the mitral valve apparatus, including the leaflets and chordae, to prevent obstruction of the valve prosthesis. Though successful at treating the primary valve pathology, the first generation mechanical prostheses were very thrombogenic and required aggressive anticoagulation. Subsequent generations of mechanical valves required less anticoagulation but still incurred a significant incidence of valve-related hemorrhage and thromboembolism. Concurrently bioprosthetic valves were being developed but long-term results in the mitral position in younger patients were disappointing, with high rates of reoperation for structural valve deterioration. Surgeons also noted that the ventricles became more spherical after removing the subvalvular apparatus and removal of the posterior leaflets and chordal structures was associated with postoperative rupture through the posterior ventricular wall. A spherical-shaped ventricle was less mechanically efficient than the normal bullet-shaped ventricle. It became evident that postoperative function was better with chordal sparing. With the development of prostheses most surgeons switched from repair to replacement. However, a few continued to develop techniques of repair. The earliest of these was a simple suture annuloplasty to reduce mitral circumference (6–8). Subsequently techniques for leaflet augmentation, repair of posterior chordae, and prosthetic ring support emerged (9,10).

The Benefits of Repair

With the availability of reliable, increasingly durable mechanical bioprostheses why pursue mitral repair? What is the justification for a procedure that might take longer, has a low but definite incidence of early failure, and requires the use of a collection of techniques to mold the valve to a successful correction?

Valve replacement is simpler, and across a population of practitioners, more consistently reliable. Mitral repair requires practice and experience to achieve consistently good results. Nevertheless, repair over forty years of progressive refinements has become amenable to more standardized proven approaches and proven to have comparable durability to replacement with a lower incidence of thromboembolism, infection, and hemorrhagic complications.

Indications for Operation

With the advent of mitral repair and its associated lower incidence of long-term complications and good long-term success, the indications for referral for mitral surgery have changed. Recent AHA/ACC guidelines suggest early intervention if repair is likely (Table 1.1) (11). Included in these recommendations is the variable of prediction of the likelihood of repair based on the surgeon's skill and experience, the disease process causing regurgitation, and the involved portions of the mitral valve. Specifically posterior leaflet prolapse due to degenerative (nonrheumatic) mitral valve disease or a ruptured chord, which is likely repairable, in contrast to involvement of the anterior leaflet, which requires a more complex repair. They emphasize that "the skill and experience of the surgeon are probably the most important determinants of whether the operation is eventually performed." Further elaborating that in general, "rheumatic and ischemic involvement of the mitral valve and calcification of the mitral valve leaflets or annulus diminish the likelihood of repair even in experienced hands."

Given these qualifications, surgery is recommended in the following scenarios: severe regurgitation with congestive heart failure symptoms and normal left ventricular function (ejection fraction > 0.60 and end-systolic dimension < 45 cm) and asymptomatic or symptomatic patients with evidence of reduced left ventricular function, specifically an ejection fraction ≤ 0.60 and/or left ventricular end-systolic dimension ≥ 45 mm, emphasizing that ejection fraction should not be allowed to fall into the low normal range, noting that there is a strong correlation of reduced survival after surgery with lower preoperative ejection fraction. If mitral repair can be accomplished in patients with a low ejection fraction, deterioration of left ventricular function can be slowed or arrested with accompanying symptomatic improvement. Shin et al. demonstrated that though ejection fraction is reduced after successful repair, stroke volume is preserved, independent of preoperative ejection fraction (12).

Surgery for mitral regurgitation is more controversial in the absence of symptoms. No data is available to recommend this, though the recent onset of atrial fibrillation is considered a relative indication, especially if there is a high likelihood of repair. The presence of atrial fibrillation for more than 1 year and/or left atrial size greater than 50 mm is a

TABLE 1.1
PERCENTAGE OF PATIENTS UNDERGOING MITRAL VALVE SURGERY WHOSE VALVES ARE REPAIRED

Indication	Class
1. Acute symptomatic MR in which repair is likely.	I
2. Patients with NYHA functional Class II, III, or IV symptoms with normal LV function defined as ejection fraction > 0.60 and end-systolic dimension < 45 mm.	I
3. Symptomatic or asymptomatic patients with mild LV dysfunction, ejection fraction 0.50 to 0.60, and end-systolic dimension 45 to 50 mm.	I
4. Symptomatic or asymptomatic patients with moderate LV dysfunction, ejection fraction 0.30 to 0.50, and/or end-systolic dimension 50 to 55 mm.	I
5. Asymptomatic patients with preserved LV function and atrial fibrillation.	IIa
6. Asymptomatic patients with preserved LV function and pulmonary hypertension (pulmonary artery systolic pressure > 50 mm Hg at rest or > 60 mm Hg with exercise).	IIa
7. Asymptomatic patients with ejection fraction 0.50 to 0.60 and end-systolic dimension < 45 mm and asymptomatic patients with ejection fraction > 0.60 and end-systolic dimension 45 to 55 mm.	IIa
8. Patients with severe LV dysfunction (ejection fraction < 0.30 and/or end-systolic dimension > 55 mm) in whom chordal preservation is highly likely.	IIa
9. Asymptomatic patients with chronic MR with preserved LV function in whom mitral valve repair is highly likely.	IIb
10. Patients with MVP* and preserved LV function who have recurrent ventricular arrhythmias despite medical therapy.	IIb
11. Asymptomatic patients with preserved LV function in whom significant doubt about the feasibility of repair exists.	III

AHA/ACC Guidelines (11)
Recommendations for Mitral Valve Surgery in Nonischemic Severe Mitral Regurgitation.
Class I: Conditions for which there is evidence and/or general agreement that a given procedure or treatment is useful and effective.
Class II: Conditions for which there is conflicting evidence and/or a divergence of opinion about the usefulness/efficacy of a procedure or treatment.
    IIa. Weight of evidence/opinion is in favor of usefulness/efficacy.
    IIb. Usefulness/efficacy is less well established by evidence/opinion.
Class III: Conditions for which there is evidence and/or general agreement that the procedure/treatment is not useful and in some cases may be harmful.
* MVP: Mitral valve prolapse

predictor of persistent atrial fibrillation after valve surgery (13). The addition of ablative operations to cure atrial fibrillation to the surgeon's armamentarium will impact this decision process, perhaps prompting earlier surgery for the combination of atrial fibrillation and mitral regurgitation.

Recently David et al. reported late outcomes of repair for floppy valves to bolster these guidelines (14). They reviewed results in 488 consecutive patients, 199 with no or minimal symptoms and 289 with symptoms at the time of surgery. With an overall survival of 61%, the survival in asymptomatic patients was 76%, identical to the age-matched general population, whereas survival for symptomatic patients was 53%, less than predicted for the general population. At 15 years, freedom from reoperation was 91%, and freedom from significant regurgitation (greater than 2+) was 85% for all, 96% for asymptomatic, and 76% for symptomatic patients. However if reoperation is the primary indicator used to assess durability, repair failure may be underreported. Flameng et al. evaluated recurrence of regurgitation as a marker instead of reoperation (15). At 8 years survival was $90.9 \pm 3.2\%$ and freedom from reoperation $94.2 \pm 2.3\%$. Rates of freedom from recurrence of nontrivial (> 1/4) and severe (> 2/4) mitral regurgitation are detailed in Table 1.2.

They calculated a linearized recurrence rate of nontrivial and severe MR of 8.3 and 3.7% per year. Excluding patients with risk factors for recurrence (chordal shortening and no annuloplasty ring or sliding plasty) the rates were 6.9 and 2.5% per year. Overall freedom from bleeding and thromboembolic events was $90.4 \pm 2.7\%$ at 8 years. They caution that durability for successful repair is not constant and should be taken into account when making surgical decisions.

When to Repair, When to Replace

Repair, in most scenarios, represents the best alternative. However, repair can be time-consuming leading to prolonged ischemic and cardiopulmonary bypass times. The decision to proceed with repair needs to be based on the likelihood of success and the long-term benefit of repair. In scenarios where the marginal benefits of repair are approximated by valve replacement, replacement may be preferable. For example, chordal sparing valve replacement provides similar mechanical advantages to repair (16) and long-term anticoagulation is not essential with a bioprosthetic valve. Replacement might be preferable in elderly patients who have no issues with durability of the prosthesis, or during emergency surgery where short ischemic time is important or repair is difficult and potentially unreliable. For example, though techniques are described to repair complete papillary muscle rupture, attempts at repair in the setting of an acute infarction are probably unwise (17). Similarly, the long-term results of repair of rheumatic valves and valves damaged by radiation (18) are significantly worse than repair for degenerative etiologies, thus rheumatic etiology might reduce the impetus for a complex repair. Durability of repair of degenerative valves can also be variable (15).

There is some objective evidence that valve repair conveys a survival benefit. Enriquez-Sarano et al. (19) compared repair to replacement for isolated mitral valve disease noting that multivariate analysis showed an independent beneficial effect of valve repair on overall and late survival, operative mortality, and postoperative ejection fraction. However, this sur-

TABLE 1.2			
RATES OF FREEDOM FROM RECURRENCE OF NONTRIVIAL AND SEVERE MITRAL REGURGITATION			
	1 Month	**5 Years**	**7 Years**
Nontrivial (> 1/4)	$94.3 \pm 1.6\%$	$58.6 \pm 4.9\%$	$27.2 \pm 8.6\%$
Severe (> 2/4)	$98.3 \pm 0.9\%$	$82.8 \pm 3.8\%$	$71.1 \pm 7.4\%$

vival benefit was not demonstrable in octogenarians (20). Gillinov et al. (21) recently compared repair to replacement for degenerative mitral disease associated with ischemic heart disease, a category perhaps often considered with ischemic mitral disease. This is a situation where many surgeons would opt for primary valve replacement, particularly in the elderly with whom a bioprosthesis can be used. Using multivariate analysis and multiphase, hazard-function analysis they determined that after 2 years repair imparted a survival advantage. Therefore every effort should be made to perform repair, even if bileaflet reconstruction is necessary. In contrast, Thourani et al. performed a retrospective case matched study in 1,250 patients, 625 mitral valve repairs matched with 625 mitral valve replacements. Repair was associated with reduced length of stay, improved in-hospital mortality, and 10-year survival, however repair did not improve 10-year survival in patients over 60 years of age or those requiring associated coronary bypass (22). This finding is at variance with other reports (23). Though results of repair are superior to replacement in all types of regurgitation not secondary to ischemic changes, the results of repair in ischemia-induced mitral regurgitation in patients over 60 are not clearly better than replacement (23). Moss et al. used propensity matching to eliminate selection bias in comparing repair and chordal sparing replacement, noting that over a median follow-up period of 3.4 years survival was better with repair but there was a trend to increased reoperation (24).

Perhaps the definitive analysis of the long-term results of mitral valve repair were published by Carpentier in 2001; the first 162 consecutive patients treated between 1970 and 1984 for mitral insufficiency secondary to nonrheumatic disease (25). The 20-year survival was similar to that for the general population, 3 patients required early reoperation and 7 required late reoperation. All 65 living patients were NYHA functional class I or II.

Interest in repair of the mitral valve has evolved over time. This is based on the problems associated with prosthetic valves including hemorrhage and thromboembolism, endocarditis, pannus formation, and structural failure. A survey of trends in valve repair from the Society of Thoracic Surgeons National Cardiac Database (NCD) demonstrated a progressive increase in the percentage of valves repaired through the 1990s (Fig. 1.1) (26).

Despite this increase, comparison with a "gold standard" suggests that repair is not being performed as often as possible. Mohty and colleagues (27) from the Mayo Clinic compared 679 repairs and 238 replacements performed between 1980 and 1995. Recognizing a referral bias (patients with a potentially repairable valve might be preferentially referred) this experience suggests a standard for rates of utilization of repair. The overall rate of repair (74%) for isolated mitral insufficiency (1980 and 1995) is almost twice that of the national rate of 42.4% in the period from 1999 and 2000 (26). Of these, 55% were repaired by annuloplasty alone with no other valvular reconstruction (26). This clearly shows that valve repair has not penetrated as much as it should.

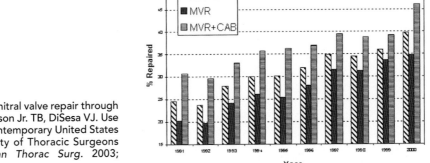

Figure 1.1   Trends in the use of mitral valve repair through the 1990s. (From Savage EB, Ferguson Jr. TB, DiSesa VJ. Use of mitral valve repair: analysis of contemporary United States experience reported to the Society of Thoracic Surgeons National Cardiac Database. *Ann Thorac Surg.* 2003; 75:820–825.)

REFERENCES

1. Little RC, Little WC. Physiological basis for mitral valve function. In: Boudoulas H, Wooley CF, eds. *Mitral Valve: Floppy Mitral Valve, Mitral Valve Prolapse, Mitral Valvular Regurgitation*. 2nd ed. Armonk: Futura Publishers; 2000:37–57.
2. Lillehei CW, Gott VL, Dewall RA, Varco RL. Surgical correction of pure mitral insufficiency by annuloplasty under direct vision. *Lancet*. 1957;1:446.
3. Merendino KA, Bruce RA: One hundred seventeen surgically treated cases of valvular rheumatic heart disease: with a preliminary report of two cases of mitral regurgitation treated under direct vision with the aid of a pump-oxygenater. *JAMA*. 1957;164:749.
4. McGoon DC. Repair of mitral insufficiency due to ruptured chordae tendineae. *J Thorac Cardiovasc Surg*. 1960; 357.
5. Starr A, Edwards ML. Mitral replacement: clinical experience with a ball valve prosthesis. *Ann Surg*. 1961;154:726.
6. Wooler GH, Nixon PG, Grinshaw VA, et al. Experiences with the repair of the mitral valve in mitral incompetence. *Thorax*. 1962;17:49.
7. Reed GE, Tice DA, Clauss RH. Asymmetric exaggerated mitral annuloplasty: repair of mitral insufficiency with hemodynamic predictability. *J Thorac Cardiovasc Surg*. 1965; 49:752.
8. Kay JH, Zubiate P, Mendez MA, et al. Mitral valve repair of significant mitral insufficiency. *Am Heart J*. 1978; 96:253.
9. Sauvage LR, Wood SJ. Technique for correction of mitral insufficiency by leaflet advancement. *J Thorac Cardiovasc Surg*. 1964 ;49:752.
10. Carpentier A, Deloche A, Dauptain J, et al. A new reconstructive operation for correction of mitral and tricuspid insufficiency. *J Thorac Cardiovasc Surg*. 1971; 61:1.
11. Bonow RO, Carabello B, de Leon AC, et al. ACC/AHA Practice Guidelines. Guidelines for the Management of Patients with Valvular Heart Disease. *Circulation*. 1998; 98:1949–1984.
12. Shin JH, Shiota T, Qin JX, et al. Forward stroke volume is preserved during left ventricular remodeling after mitral valve repair. *J Am Coll Cardiol*. 2003; 41(6 Suppl B):515.
13. Betriu A, Chaitman BR, Almazan A, et al. Preoperative determinants of return to sinus rhythm after valve replacement. In: Cohn LH, Gallucci V, eds. *Cardiac Bioprostheses*. New York: Yorke Medical Books; 1982:184.
14. David TE, Ivanov J, Armstrong S, Rakowski H. Late outcomes of mitral valve repair for floppy valves: implications for asymptomatic patients. *J Thorac Cardiovasc Surg*. 2003:125:1143–1152.
15. Flameng W, Herijgers P, Bogaerts K. Recurrence of mitral valve regurgitation after mitral valve repair in degenerative valve disease. *Circulation*. 2003;107:1609–1613.
16. Komeda M, David TE, Rao V, et al. Late hemodynamic effects of the preserved papillary muscles during mitral valve replacement. *Circulation*. 1994; 90:II190–194.
17. Tavakoli R, Weber A, Brunner-La Rocca H, et al. Results of surgery for irreversible moderate to severe mitral valve regurgitation secondary to myocardial infarction. *Eur J Cardiothorac Surg*. 2002; 21:818–824.
18. Crestanello JA, McGregor CG, Danielson GK, et al. Mitral and tricuspid valve repair in patients with previous mediastinal radiation therapy. *Ann Thorac Surg*. 2004; 78:826–831.
19. Enriquez-Sarano M, Schaff HV, Orszulak TA, et al. Valve repair improves the outcome of surgery for mitral regurgitation. A multivariate analysis. *Circulation*. 1995; 91:1022–1028.
20. DiGregorio V, Zehr KJ, Orszulak TA et al. Results of mitral surgery in octogenarians with isolated nonrheumatic mitral regurgitation. *Ann Thorac Surg*. 2004; 78:807–813.
21. Gillinov AM, Faber C, Houghtaling PL, et al. Repair versus replacement for degenerative mitral valve disease with coexisting ischemic heart disease. *J Thorac Cardiovasc Surg*. 2003; 125:1350–1362.
22. Thourani VH, Weintraub WS, Guyton RA, et al. Outcomes and long-term survival for patients undergoing mitral valve repair versus replacement: effect of age and concomitant coronary artery bypass grafting. *Circulation*. 2003; 108:298–304.
23. Enriquez-Sarano M, Schaff HV, Frye RL. Mitral regurgitation: what causes the leakage is fundamental to the outcome of valve repair. *Circulation*. 2003; 108:253–256.
24. Moss RR, Humphries KH, Gao M, et al. Outcome of mitral valve repair or replacement: a comparison by propensity score analysis. *Circulation*. 2003; 108 Suppl 1:II90-7.
25. Braunberger E, Deloche A, Berrebi A, et al. Very long-term results (more than 20 years) of valve repair with Carpentier's techniques in nonrheumatic mitral valve insufficiency. *Circulation*. 2001; 104:I8–11.
26. Savage EB, Ferguson Jr. TB, DiSesa VJ. Use of mitral valve repair: analysis of contemporary United States experience reported to the Society of Thoracic Surgeons National Cardiac Database. *Ann Thorac Surg*. 2003; 75:820–825.
27. Mohty, D, Orszulak, TA, Schaff, HV, et al. Very long-term survival and durability of mitral valve repair for mitral valve prolapse. *Circulation*. 2001; 104:I-1–7.

Functional Anatomy of the Mitral Valve

OVERVIEW

Historically, the mitral valve is described as composed of the leaflets, chordae, and papillary muscles. However, the mitral valve structurally and functionally is part of the left ventricle and intimately associated with the atrium and fibrous skeleton of the heart. Thus, alterations to the fibrous skeleton and ventricular and atrial muscle contribute to and affect valvular function.

LEAFLETS

The leaflets are the valve component that creates the division between the atrium and ventricle. There are two distinct leaflets: the anterior or aortic and posterior or mural. The anterior leaflet is usually comprised of a single trapezoidal-shaped unit. The posterior leaflet is punctuated with multiple slits and clefts that define usually three, but up to six, distinct scallops (Fig. 2.1)

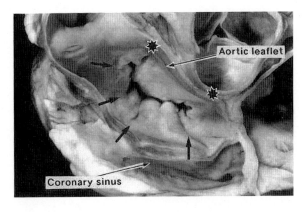

Figure 2.1 Photograph of the mitral valve. Note multiple clefts in the posterior leaflet (*arrows*). (From Angelini A, Ho SY, Thiene G, Anderson RH. Anatomy of the mitral valve. In: Boudoulas H, Wooley CF, eds. *Mitral Valve: Floppy Mitral Valve, Mitral Valve Prolapse, Mitral Valvular Regurgitation.* 2nd ed. Armonk: Futura Publishers; 2000:9.)

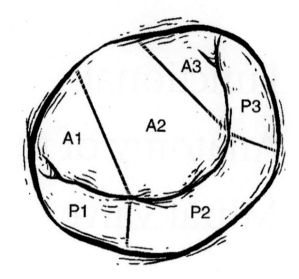

Figure 2.2   Segments of the mitral valve. (From Kouchoukos NT, Blackstone EH, Doty DB, Hanley FL, Karp RB. *Kirklin/Barratt-Boyes Cardiac Surgery: Morphology, Diagnostic Criteria, Natural History, Techniques, Results, and Indications.* Philadelphia: Churchill Livingstone; 2003:21.)

(though often not depicted this way in line drawings in texts). The anterior and posterior leaflets are separated at the commissures but there is usually some continuity of the valve tissue close to the annulus. Further, if one looks at the chordal distribution, at the commissures, chordae are distributed to both leaflets from a common structural source—so the leaflets form a single functional unit. Nevertheless, it is useful for the purposes of valve repair to differentiate anterior from posterior. However, one must remember that multiple separately suspended distinct units come together to make the valve competent. To describe components of mitral valve repair it is useful to label the scallops by position (Fig. 2.2); posteriorly from left to right P1, P2, P3, with corresponding regions of the anterior leaflet A1, A2, and A3 (1,2).

When in the closed position, the orifice is obscured by the anterior and posterior leaflets. The anterior comprises about one half to two thirds of this area, the posterior comprises about one third to one half of this area. The point of attachment of the anterior leaflet comprises one third of the circumference of the annulus (the fibrous area) and the posterior leaflets comprises two thirds of the circumference of the annulus (the muscular area). The fibrous support of the anterior leaflet is fixed, the muscular support of the posterior leaflet can enlarge and does so when annular dilatation is associated with mitral regurgitation. The leaflets themselves are comprised of clear and rough zones (Fig. 2.3). The clear zone is between the line of closure and the annulus and can be quite thin, almost transparent. The rough zone extends from the line of closure to the free edge, characterized by thicker, nodular ridges which promote sealing of the orifice on valve closure (3).

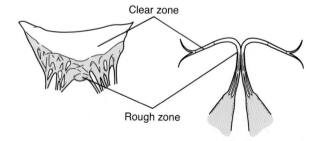

Figure 2.3   Zones of the mitral leaflets. (From Seccombe JF, Schaff HV. Mitral valve repair: current techniques and indications. In: Franco KL, Verrier ED, eds. *Advanced Therapy in Cardiac Surgery.* St. Louis: B.C. Decker; 1999:222.)

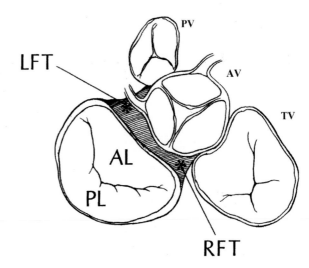

Figure 2.4   Relational anatomy of the mitral valve. LFT and RFT, left and right fibrous trigones; AL and PL, anterior and posterior mitral leaflets; PV, AV, and TV, pulmonic, aortic, and tricuspid valves. (From Chitwood Jr. WR. Mitral valve repair: ischemic. In: Kaiser LR, Kron IL, Spray TL. *Mastery of Cardiothoracic Surgery*. Philadelphia: Lippincott-Raven Publishers; 1998:310.)

ANNULUS

Of the four heart valves, the mitral valve is the only valve that has a distinguishable annulus. However, the presence of a fibrous annular structure is variable and discontinuous. The firmest site of support for the mitral valve is the region of fibrous continuity between the aortic and mitral valves, the extent of which is delineated by the right and left fibrous trigones (Fig. 2.4). Nevertheless, for surgical purposes, the annulus is considered the area of attachment of the valve leaflets to the atrial muscle. The annulus is a functional component of the mitral valve. The annulus is quite flexible and changes shape throughout the cardiac cycle (4). With normal systolic function, the annulus will reduce in size by 20% to 40%.

Saddle Shape

Functionally the mitral annulus is not two-dimensional but in fact three-dimensional assuming a saddle shape (Fig. 2.5) (5). The curvature imposed by the saddle shape reduces mechanical stress on the leaflets. The curvature of the saddle shape or height of the "saddle horn" is reduced in a model of ischemic mitral regurgitation (6). This may have implications in choosing techniques for annular reduction and stabilization.

TENDINOUS CHORDS

The tendinous chords, as functional extensions of the papillary muscles, perform the dual function of maintaining valvular competence by preventing leaflet prolapse and maintaining ventricular geometry by providing cross-ventricular support. The chords originate from the apical portions of the papillary muscles or directly from the posterior ventricular wall. They insert either into the free edge of the leaflets or on their ventricular surface. Chords

Figure 2.5   Shape of the human mitral annulus. Fourier smoothed reconstruction from images obtained by transesophageal echocardiography. The commissures are located at the low points of the saddle. (From Salgo IS, Gorman JH 3rd, Gorman RC, et al. Effect of annular shape on leaflet curvature in reducing mitral leaflet stress. *Circulation*. 2002; 106:711–717.)

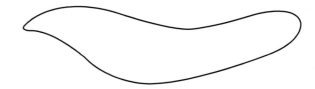

have been characterized a number of ways. The most useful for repair purposes is to describe the first-degree chords as those inserting into the valve edge and the second-degree chords as those inserting into the underside of the leaflet. Both first-degree and second-degree chords originate from the papillary muscles and third-degree chords originate from the ventricular wall and insert into the base of the posterior leaflet.

PAPILLARY MUSCLES

There are two papillary muscles associated with the mitral valve. When looking from the atrial side, the anterolateral is to the left and the posteromedial is to the right. The muscles are located under their respective commissures. They originate from the lower third of the left ventricular free wall. The papillary muscles are extensions of the ventricular muscle from which they originate. The chords originate from the fibrous tips of these muscles, extending to insert on the mitral leaflets. The blood supply of the anterolateral papillary muscle derives from the left circumflex and/or diagonal systems. The blood supply of the posteromedial papillary muscle derives from the posterolateral coronary branches whether it originates from the left or right coronary system. The papillary muscles adjust tension and stabilize the valve during the cardiac cycle, rather than pulling the chords and leaflets into position. The function of the papillary muscles and their position is greatly dependent on the status of the ventricular myocardium underlying it. Displacement of the papillary muscle by distorted ventricular geometry is one mechanism for the creation of mitral regurgitation.

REFERENCES

1. Kumar N, Kumar M, Duran CM. A revised terminology for recording surgical findings of the mitral valve. *J Heart Valve Disease.* 1995; 4:70.
2. Kouchoukos NT, Blackstone EH, Doty DB, Hanley FL, Karp RB. Kirklin/Barratt-Boyes cardiac surgery: morphology, diagnostic criteria, natural history, techniques, results, and indications. Philadelphia: Churchill Livingstone, 2003:19–21.
3. Seccombe JF, Schaff HV. Mitral valve repair: current techniques and indications. In: Franco KL, Verrier ED, eds. *Advanced Therapy in Cardiac Surgery*, St. Louis: B.C. Decker; 1999:220–231.
4. Komoda T, Hetzer R, Oellinger J, et al. Mitral annular flexibility. *J Card Surg.* 1997; 12:102–109.
5. Salgo IS, Gorman JH 3rd, Gorman RC, et al. Effect of annular shape on leaflet curvature in reducing mitral leaflet stress. *Circulation.* 2002; 106:711–717.
6. Tibayan FA, Rodriguez F, Langer F, et al. Annular remodeling in chronic ischemic mitral regurgitation: ring selection implications. *Ann Thorac Surg.* 2003; 76:1549–1554.

Pathology of Mitral Valve Disease

CLASSIFICATION OF THE PATHOLOGIC PROCESSES THAT CAUSE MITRAL REGURGITATION

The pathologic processes that lead to mitral regurgitation include degenerative valve processes (fibroelastic deficiency, rheumatic valvulitis, myxomatous [Barlow's] disease and Marfan's syndrome) (1), congenital malformation, destruction by endocarditis, and ischemic dysfunction. Carpentier noted that though the etiology of regurgitation may vary, the approach to repair is based on the valvular deformity caused by the deformative process. Treating regurgitation based on the deformity is called the "functional approach" (2). The goal of the functional approach is to restore normal function rather than anatomy. This points to a final common pathway for mitral regurgitation—the initial abnormality leads to regurgitation, which promotes ventricular and annular dilatation, worsening the regurgitation.

The three types of abnormalities are based on the positions of the leaflets during valve closure (Fig. 3.1). In Type I, the leaflets are in normal position relative to the annulus. This is usually associated with normal or abnormal leaflets, and the regurgitation is a result of a hole in the leaflet, central regurgitation secondary to annular dilation, leaflet abnormalities preventing proper leaflet coaptation, or a combination of these abnormalities. In a Type II abnormality, one or both of the leaflets prolapses relative to the valvular plane. This is due to papillary muscle or chordal rupture; or elongation or redundancy of the body of the leaflet. Type III abnormalities are related to restricted leaflet motion. The restriction prevents leaflet coaptation. This can be due to leaflet abnormalities, such as thickening or commissural fusion; chordal abnormalities, including fusion and thickening; papillary muscle contraction; or ventricular abnormalities, such as scarring or dilatation. In Type IIIa the motion of one or both leaflets is restricted throughout the cardiac cycle secondary to rheumatic changes. In Type IIIb the motion of one or both leaflets is restricted during systole secondary to papillary muscle displacement (1).

FIBROELASTIC DEFICIENCY

Fibroelastic deficiency occurs mostly in the elderly with a short history of valvular dysfunction. The leaflets are transparent, and except for the prolapsing segment there is no excess tissue. The chordae are thin, fragile, and elongated. The annulus is dilated and often infiltrated with calcium (1).

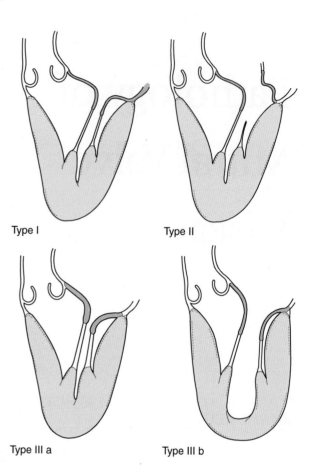

Type I   Type II

Type III a   Type III b

Figure 3.1 Carpentier's functional classification is based on the opening and closing motions of the mitral leaflets. Type I has normal motion of the leaflets and mitral regurgitation is on the basis of the leaflet perforation or annular dilatation. In Type II dysfunction (increased leaflet motion) the free edge of the leaflet travels above the plane of the mitral annulus during systole due to chordal elongation or rupture. Type IIIa dysfunction implies restricted opening leaflet motion during diastole and systole due to rheumatic changes. Type IIIb dysfunction correlates to restricted leaflet motion during systole secondary to papillary muscle displacement. (From Adams DH, Fisoufi F. Another chapter in an enlarging book: repair degenerative mitral valves. *J Thorac Cardiovasc Surg.* 2003; 125:1197–1199.)

MYXOMATOUS MITRAL VALVE DISEASE (BARLOW'S DISEASE)

Myxomatous disease of the mitral valve generally appears early in life. Patients present with a prolonged history of a murmur, thickened leaflets, substantial excess tissue, and a dilated annulus, which may be calcified (1). Chordae may be elongated and thinned. Often isolated ruptures are present, contributing to the focal prolapse. Classically, the most common abnormality is focal enlargement of the posterior central scallop (P2) with an associated ruptured chorda. Mills et al. comparing unileaflet versus bileaflet prolapse, found that patients with unileaflet prolapse were younger and had a higher incidence of flail leaflets (3). Patients with bileaflet prolapse were less likely to be hypertensive and had mechanically stronger chordae though leaflet strength was similar to patients with unileaflet prolapse.

MARFAN'S SYNDROME

Marfan's syndrome of the mitral valve is characterized by excess tissue, thickened leaflets, and a dilated annulus (1).

RHEUMATIC MITRAL VALVE DISEASE

Rheumatic disease of the mitral valve more commonly results in stenosis than regurgitation. However, regurgitation can occur with or without associated stenosis. Leaflets become thickened and stiff, and can be calcified. Annular calcification is also common. In contrast to other disease processes chordae become thickened and foreshortened and fuse together.

Chordal rupture is uncommon. The foreshortened chordae pull the leaflets towards the papillary muscle tips, restricting ventricular enlargement during ventricular relaxation.

ISCHEMIC MITRAL VALVE DISEASE

Ischemia-related mitral regurgitation represents a spectrum of disease processes often lumped together into a single group for analysis. Acute ischemia can result in mitral regurgitation, which often resolves over time. However, mitral regurgitation accompanying acute myocardial infarction worsens long-term prognosis, increasing mortality (4). Implications, safety of surgery, and likelihood of repair differ greatly based on the time and type of presentation. In most cases, the anatomic substrate of the valve itself is normal; the leaflets bear no structural defects, the chords are not elongated or ruptured, and the annulus is not dilated. Acutely the defect in valvular competence is related to the changed relationships of the structures supporting the valve, specifically the infarcted myocardial wall causes apical displacement of the leaflets and abnormal tethering, causing leaflet deformation and preventing proper coaptation (5,6). In contrast to regurgitation secondary to dilated cardiomyopathy, which is associated with symmetrical mitral valve deformation (Fig. 3.2), mitral valve deformation is asymmetric with an ischemic cardiomyopathy (7). Timek et al. demonstrated, in a sheep model of ischemic mitral regurgitation, that proximal left circumflex coronary artery occlusion causes central and holosystolic regurgitation, by delaying valve closure, increasing mitral annular area and displacing both papillary muscle tips away from the septal annulus at end systole (8).

The concept of papillary muscle dysfunction as a cause of mitral regurgitation is simplified and incorrect. In dogs, isolated papillary muscle infarction does not cause regurgitation, instead the infarction of the supporting wall leads to malposition and abnormal motion of the papillary muscle (9). Tibayan et al. observed in a sheep model that ischemic changes included septal-lateral dilatation and lateral displacement of the posterior papillary muscle (10), and Lai et al. observed malcoaptation of the posterior leaflet scallops, suggesting all of these changes be addressed during repair (11). One approach is to undersize the valve to improve long-term results (12).

As described above, ischemic mitral regurgitation results from tethering, however ischemic mitral regurgitation can also be secondary to abnormal scarring and healing, specifically the papillary muscle can elongate or rupture, causing prolapse instead of regurgitation (Fig. 3.3).

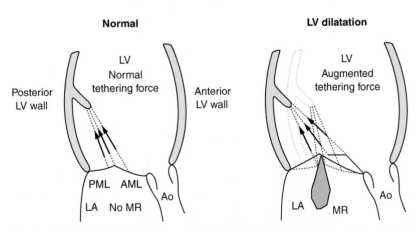

Figure 3.2 Mechanical and geometric changes that lead to ischema-induced mitral regurgitation. (From Kumanohoso T, Otsuji Y, Yoshifuku S, et al. Mechanism of higher incidence of ischemic mitral regurgitation in patients with inferior myocardial infarction: quantitative analysis of left ventricular and mitral valve geometry in 103 patients with prior myocardial infarction. *J Thorac Cardiovasc Surg.* 2003; 125:135–143.)

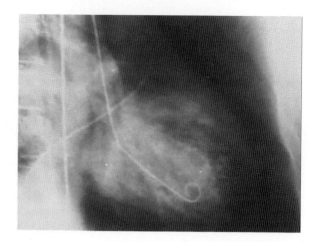

Figure 3.3   Ischemic cardiomyopathy: Angiogram demonstrating a low ejection fraction and severe mitral regurgitation. (Clip 1, Case 2)

Acute vs. Chronic Regurgitation

The scenario of presentation has significant implication in the approach to ischemia-related mitral regurgitation. In the acute situation after myocardial infarction, the principle cause of regurgitation is tethering. There is no associated annular dilation. Therefore, repair in the acute situation is difficult and replacement is often necessary. Often regurgitation in the peri-infarct period will improve spontaneously or with revascularization. If possible a delay in operation may be advisable to avoid valve replacement.

Papillary Muscle Rupture

A small subset of patients develops mitral regurgitation secondary to partial or complete rupture of the infarcted papillary muscle. As the papillary muscle has multiple heads, the rupture can involve a single head, multiple heads, or the whole muscle. The level of symptoms will be related to the degree of regurgitation predating the rupture, the change in the degree of regurgitation with the rupture, and the extent of the associated infarction. Complete rupture is generally very poorly tolerated and must be addressed emergently. Complete rupture with extensive necrosis may best be treated with chordal-sparing valve replacement (13).

Rupture of the posterior papillary muscle is five times more common than rupture of the anterior muscle (14). This is based on the blood supply to the papillary muscle. The supply to the anterior papillary muscle comes from dual sources. The supply to the posterior papillary muscle comes from a single source.

REFERENCES

1. Adams DH, Fisoufi F. Another chapter in an enlarging book: repair degenerative mitral valves. *J Thorac Cardiovasc Surg.* 2003; 125:1197–1199.
2. Carpentier A. Cardiac valve surgery—the "French Correction." *J Thorac Cardiovasc Surg.* 1983; 86:323–337.
3. Mills WR, Barber JE, Skiles JA. Clinical, echocardiographic, and biomechanical differences in mitral valve prolapse affecting one or both leaflets. *Am J Cardiol.* 2002; 89; 1394–1399.
4. Lamas GA, Mitchell GF, Flaker GC, et al. Clinical significance of mitral regurgitation after acute myocardial infarction. Survival and ventricular enlargement investigators. *Circulation.* 1997; 96:827–833.
5. Levine RA, Hung J, Otsuji Y, et al. Mechanistic insights into functional mitral regurgitation. *Curr Cardiol Rep.* 2002; 4:125–129.
6. Kumanohoso T, Otsuji Y, Yoshifuku S, et al. Mechanism of higher incidence of ischemic mitral regurgitation in patients with inferior myocardial infarction: quantitative analysis of left ventricular and mitral valve geometry in 103 patients with prior myocardial infarction. *J Thorac Cardiovasc Surg.* 2003; 125:135–143.
7. Kwan J, Shiota T, Agler DA, et al. Geometric differences of the mitral apparatus between ischemic and dilated cardiomyopathy with significant mitral regurgitation. Real-time three-dimensional echocardiography study. *Circulation.* 2003; 107:1135–1140.
8. Timek TA, Lai DT, Tibayan F, et al. Ischemia in three left ventricular regions: insights into the pathogenesis of acute ischemic mitral regurgitation. *J Thorac Cardiovasc Surg.* 2003; 125:559–569.
9. Kisslo JA. (Personal Communication)

10. Tibayan FA, Rodriguez F, Zasio MK, et al. Geometric distortions of the mitral valvular-ventricular complex in chronic ischemic mitral regurgitation. *Circulation*. 2003; 108 Suppl 1:II116–21.
11. Lai DT, Tibayan FA, Myrmel T, et al. Mechanistic insights into posterior mitral leaflet inter-scallop malcoaptation during acute ischemic mitral regurgitation. *Circulation*. 2002; 106:I40–I45.
12. Enriquez-Sarano M, Schaff HV, Frye RL. Mitral regurgitation: what causes the leakage is fundamental to the outcome of valve repair. *Circulation*. 2003; 108:253–256.
13. David TE. Techniques and results of mitral valve repair for ischemic mitral regurgitation. *J Card Surg*. 1994; 9:274–277.
14. Chitwood WR. Mitral valve repair: ischemic. In: Kaiser LR, Kron IL, Spray TL. *Mastery of Cardiothoracic Surgery*. Philadelphia: Lippincott-Raven, 1998:309–321.

Assessing the Functional Substrate of Mitral Regurgitation with Echocardiography

4

Echocardiography, in particular transesophageal echocardiography (TEE) has emerged as the preferred method for the assessment and quantification of the nature and degree of mitral regurgitation. Complete assessment of the mitral valve is possible with details of structure and function easily observed. The results of this assessment will guide the surgeon and the referring physician. Points of assessment include the degree of regurgitation; the valvular abnormality, indicating the likelihood for repair; the degree of ventricular dysfunction; pulmonary pressure; and the status of other valves.

A good transthoracic echocardiogram (TTE) is often adequate for assessment; however, any remaining questions should be clarified by transesophageal echocardiogram (TEE). In one series of 118 patients comparing TTE to TEE, 25% had mitral regurgitation detected by transesophageal echocardiography that was not noted by transthoracic echocardiography; of these 14% had significant (2 to 3+) mitral regurgitation (1). TEE also can demonstrate specific abnormalities, such as a ruptured chordae, which may not be detected with TTE.

TEE is uniquely useful for intraoperative assessment of the mitral valve. It should be used for a final assessment before surgery begins and after the completion of the repair. Multiple views of the valve from different angles provide systematic assessment of the mitral valve. These views are detailed in Figure 4.1.

Functional analysis is provided by pulsed, continuous, and color flow Doppler. Pulsed-wave Doppler measures velocity at a specific point but has a limited velocity range; it is useful for measuring pulmonary venous flow. Continuous Doppler is limited by spatial ambiguity but has a greater velocity range; it is useful for measuring high velocity flow through a stenotic valve. Color-flow mapping is used to assess patterns of blood flow (2). In color-flow Doppler, flow towards the transducer is red and flow away from the transducer is blue. Higher velocities are represented by brighter hues.

Doppler color-flow imaging is used to assess the degree of mitral regurgitation. The size of the jet indexed to the size of the atrium provides a consistent accurate assessment, though there are exceptions. Peripheral jets or jets next to the wall will recruit less blood, therefore, they may be judged as smaller unless appropriately corrected. With moderate-to-severe regurgitation flow reversal can be noted in the pulmonary veins (3). Effective regurgitant

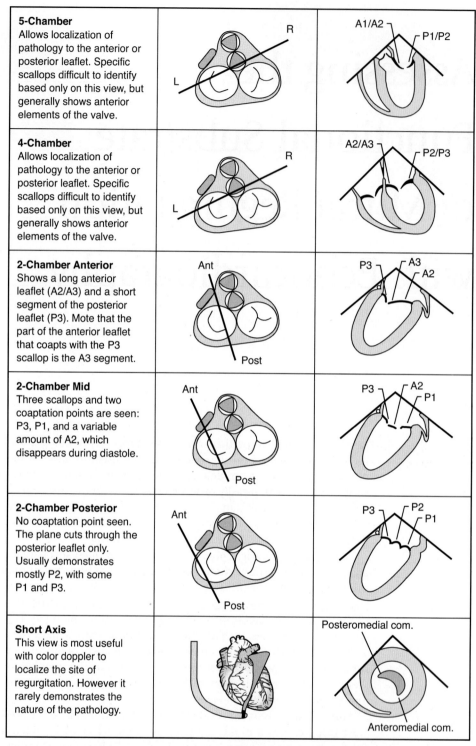

5-Chamber Allows localization of pathology to the anterior or posterior leaflet. Specific scallops difficult to identify based only on this view, but generally shows anterior elements of the valve.		
4-Chamber Allows localization of pathology to the anterior or posterior leaflet. Specific scallops difficult to identify based only on this view, but generally shows anterior elements of the valve.		
2-Chamber Anterior Shows a long anterior leaflet (A2/A3) and a short segment of the posterior leaflet (P3). Mote that the part of the anterior leaflet that coapts with the P3 scallop is the A3 segment.		
2-Chamber Mid Three scallops and two coaptation points are seen: P3, P1, and a variable amount of A2, which disappears during diastole.		
2-Chamber Posterior No coaptation point seen. The plane cuts through the posterior leaflet only. Usually demonstrates mostly P2, with some P1 and P3.		
Short Axis This view is most useful with color doppler to localize the site of regurgitation. However it rarely demonstrates the nature of the pathology.		

Figure 4.1   Views obtained by transesophageal echocardiography. (From Lambert AS, Miller JP, Merrick SH, et al. Improved evaluation of the location and mechanism of mitral valve regurgitation with a systematic transesophageal echocardiography examination. *Anesth Analg.* 1999; 88:1205–1212.)

orifice area calculated on the basis of the proximal isovelocity surface area method has been advocated as an accurate, consistent method of assessment (4). Central jets imply annular dilatation with resultant poor leaflet coaptation, eccentric jets imply leaflet pathology with the jet directed away from the affected leaflet.

The severity of regurgitation is judged by the proportion of the maximal area of the jet relative to the left atrium; 1%–15%, (1+); 16%–35%, (2+); 36%–55%, (3+); and greater than 55%, (4+). The severity of regurgitation is also assessed by the direction of flow in the pulmonary veins; blunted or reversed flow implies greater degrees of regurgitation. These terms are relative; though one laboratory may report 1+ as mild, 2+ as moderate, 3+ as moderately severe, and 4+ as severe, semantics vary and should be clarified before making management decisions (5). Assessment can be quite subjective and is operator dependent, many of the settings on the machine (e.g., gain) can make the degree of regurgitation seem greater or less than it really is. Likewise the size of the atrium will have an impact on the relative assessment of regurgitant jets and pulmonary venous flow.

The other factor that impacts greatly on the degree of regurgitation is peripheral vascular resistance; this is specifically reflected by the systolic blood pressure. At lower blood pressures, particularly after the induction of anesthesia, the degree of regurgitation may be underestimated. At higher blood pressures, particularly in patients who presents with poorly controlled hypertension, the degree of regurgitation may be overestimated. Thus knowledge of the blood pressure at the time of assessment is useful. Intraoperatively, the blood pressure needs to be artificially raised to completely assess the competency of the valve. This can be done with an infusion of phenylephrine to raise the systolic BP to 150 mmHg.

As three-dimensional echocardiography improves, the pictures showing the dynamic valvular pathology will help in planning reparative procedures (Figs. 4.2–4.6).

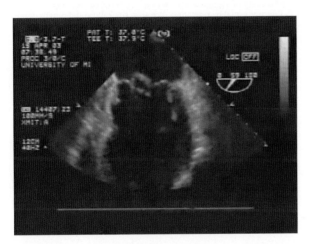

Figure 4.2   Preoperative echocardiogram of a myxomatous valve with a flail posterior leaflet and anteriorly directed jet. (Clip 1, Case 1)

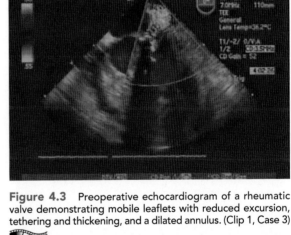

Figure 4.3   Preoperative echocardiogram of a rheumatic valve demonstrating mobile leaflets with reduced excursion, tethering and thickening, and a dilated annulus. (Clip 1, Case 3)

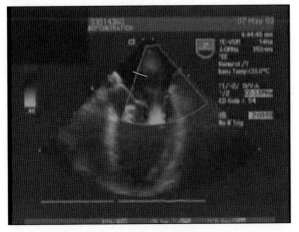

Figure 4.4   Preoperative echocardiogram of a myxomatous valve with anterior leaflet prolapse and a posteriorly directed jet. (Clip 1, Case 4)

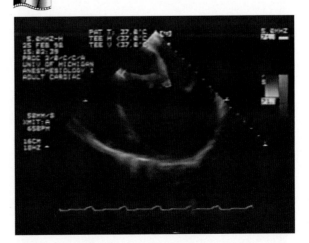

Figure 4.5   Preoperative echocardiogram of mitral regurgitation secondary to a dilated cardiomyopathy (Clip 1, Case 5)

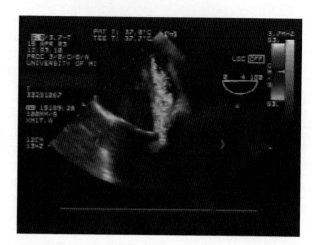

Figure 4.6 Preoperative echocardiogram of mitral regurgitation secondary to chronic ischemia demonstrating a dilated annulus, tethered chords, and poor coaptation (Clip 2, Case 2)

REFERENCES

1. Castello R, Fagan L Jr, Lenzen P, Pearson AC, Labovitz AJ. Comparison of transthoracic and transesophageal echocardiography for assessment of left-sided valvular regurgitation. *Am J Cardiol.* 1991; 68:1677–1680.
2. Kodavatiganti R: Intraoperative assessment of the mitral valve by transesophageal echocardiography: an overview. *Ann Cardiac Anaesthesia.* 2002; 5:127–134.
3. Enriquez-Sarano M, Dujardin KS, Tribouilloy CM, et al. Determinants of pulmonary venous flow reversal in mitral regurgitation and its usefulness in determining the severity of regurgitation. *Am J Cardiol.* 1999; 83:535–541.
4. Enriquez-Sarano M, Miller FA Jr, Hayes SN, et al. Effective mitral regurgitant orifice area: clinical use and pitfalls of the proximal isovelocity surface area method. *J Am Coll Cardiol.* 1995; 25:703–709.
5. Muehrcke DD, Cosgrove DM. Mitral valvuloplasty. In Edmunds, LH Jr., ed. *Cardiac Surgery in the Adult.* New York: McGraw-Hill, 1997:998.

Overview of Mitral Valve Repair

5

PREOPERATIVE AND PERIOPERATIVE ASSESSMENT

Details of the assessment of the mitral valve with echocardiography are reviewed in Chapter 4. It is important to review the echocardiogram prior to beginning the operative procedure. The echocardiogram will provide dynamic details about the abnormality of the valve that are unavailable with the heart arrested, such as which leaflet prolapses—the posterior, the anterior, or both? Does the whole leaflet prolapse or part of the leaflet? Where is the jet, central or lateral? Which direction is the jet positioned? Anteriorly—suggesting posterior-leaflet pathology, or posteriorly—suggesting anterior leaflet pathology. Are their ruptured chords? Is the annulus dilated? Is there calcification in the annulus or leaflet? Is leaflet motion restricted? This provides valuable information when deciding how to complete the repair.

An important area to focus on is the location and degree of prolapse. The anterior leaflet is considered to prolapse if it protrudes above the annular plane during systole. When assessing the anterior leaflet in the flaccid arrested heart it will always appear to prolapse, emphasizing the value of reviewing the echocardiogram.

Once the heart is arrested and the atrium is opened, inspection of the atrium and valvular structures will determine the necessary components of the repair. Adequate visualization of the valve is important. The mitral valve can be approached via transseptal or right lateral approaches. Visualization via the lateral approach is facilitated by dissection of the intraatrial groove.

Jet lesions in the atrium can direct attention to the site of abnormality. Hooks allow examination of the leaflets and subvalvular apparatus for mobility and integrity. Classifying the leaflet abnormality as Types I, II, or III will also guide the repair (Figs. 5.1–5.7).

GENERAL PRINCIPLES OF REPAIR

The goal of the various repair techniques is to identify the abnormality causing the leak then repair or compensate for the abnormality. Ideally correct application of repair techniques will produce appropriate coaptation. The rough zones of the leaflet should be in contact. The ratio of leaflet surface area to valve orifice area should be corrected to its natural 2:1 ratio. Because annular dilatation is a component of chronic mitral regurgitation, some type of annular support is necessary. Annuloplasty often completes the repair but cannot compensate for an inadequate repair.

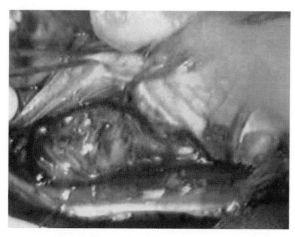

Figure 5.1 Dissection of the intraatrial groove. (Clip 2, Case 5)

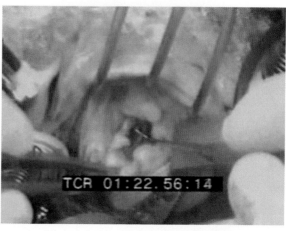

Figure 5.2 Intraoperative evaluation demonstrating a myxomatous valve with bileaflet proplapse and posterior stretched chords. . (Clip 1, Case 6)

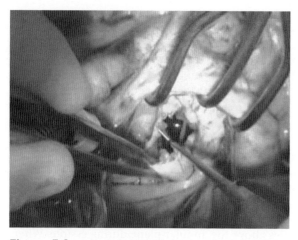

Figure 5.3 Intraoperative evaluation demonstrating a myxomatous valve with a posterior flail leaflet and ruptured chords to P2 and a P1-P2 cleft. (Clip 2, Case 1)

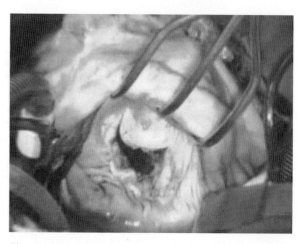

Figure 5.4 Intraoperative evaluation demonstrating a rheumatic valve with stiff leaflets, commissural and cleft fusion, and thickened, shortened chords. (Clip 2, Case 3)

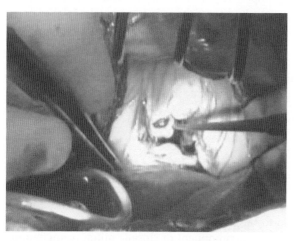

Figure 5.5 Intraoperative evaluation demonstrating anterior leaflet prolapse. (Clip 2, Case 4)

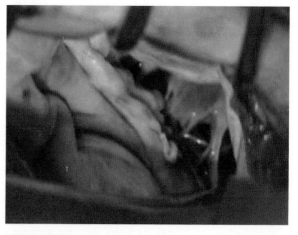

Figure 5.6 Intraoperative evaluation demonstrating normal leaflet structure and a dilated annulus. (Clip 3, Case 2)

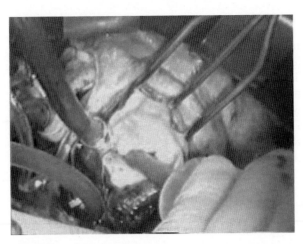

Figure 5.7 Intraoperative evaluation demonstrating a normal appearing valve with a dilated annulus. (Clip 3, Case 5)

Sequence of Repair

In general, sequential performance of the components of repair should be logical with previous steps supporting subsequent steps. After analyzing the defects and deciding on the necessary components, placement of the sutures that will be used to secure the annuloplasty ring will help bring the valve into view. Leaflet components should be repaired before performing procedures to secure leaflet excursion. Securing the ring in place prior to tying artificial chordae will allow for more accurate length determination.

Suture Material and Placement

For suturing the leaflets, fine 4-0 monofilament suture (e.g., polypropylene) has been recommended. However, Lim et al. reported reoperation necessitated by perforation of the apposing leaflet by the stiff tail of a polypropylene suture used for a previous leaflet repair (1). They recommend using a soft braided suture (e.g., polyester) for leaflet repair. For insertion of the annuloplasty ring or band 2-0 braided polyester sutures are adequate. For artificial chordae 2-0, 4-0, or 5-0 Goretex is recommended. One author considers 5-0 too weak and prone to rupture.

GENERAL PRINCIPLES FOR CLOSURE OF LEAFLET DEFECTS

Whether closing a gap at the commissure or between scallops or closing a defect after leaflet excision, the suture repair must be strong and must not distort the leaflet anatomy. The sturdiness of the tissue is very important. Thin tissue will not hold sutures and will easily tear. Avoid creating pleats in the valve tissue and foreshortening it by using an interrupted or a running-locking suture (Fig. 5.8). An additional advantage of a running-locking suture is to avoid knots at the site of leaflet apposition.

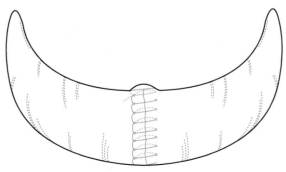

Figure 5.8 Running-locking suture to prevent crimping along the suture line. The suture is started at the edge and tied on the ventricular side of the leaflet, then brought up through the atrial side. Sutures are placed horizontally, locking the previous loop then pulled up and set before the next suture bite is taken.

One-Leaflet versus Two-Leaflet Repair

The goal of the classic principles of mitral valve repair outlined above is to create two functional leaflets. Specifically if both leaflets prolapse then reparative techniques must be applied to both. Another alternative is to simplify the task by repairing the posterior leaflet to function as a buttress for the anterior leaflet, creating a functional unileaflet valve. This concept was specifically addressed by Gillinov et al., examining the outcomes in patients who had bileaflet prolapse with no chordal abnormalities (rupture or elongation) that underwent isolated posterior-leaflet repair and annuloplasty (2). This approach was preferentially used in 93 patients with excellent long-term results (3).

REFERENCES

1. Lam BK, Gillinov AM, Cosgrove DM 3rd. Failed mitral valve repair caused by polypropylene suture. *Ann Thorac Surg.* 2003; 76:1716–1717.
2. Gillinov AM, Cosgrove DM 3rd, Wahi S, et al. Is anterior leaflet repair always necessary in repair of bileaflet mitral valve prolapse? *Ann Thorac Surg.* 1999; 68:820–823.
3. Cho L, Gillinov AM, Cosgrove DM 3rd, et al. Echocardiographic assessment of the mechanisms of correction of bileaflet prolapse causing mitral regurgitation with only posterior leaflet repair surgery. *Am J Cardiol.* 2000 Dec 15; 86(12):1349–1351.

Annuloplasty: Sutures, Bands, and Rings

6

ROLE AND APPLICATION OF ANNULOPLASTY

An annuloplasty is usually required to create proper leaflet apposition and prevent recurrent annular dilatation because annular dilatation is common to most cases of chronic mitral regurgitation (1). The aim is to remodel the annulus to a systolic shape. Cohn reported that the use of an annuloplasty ring was significantly associated with a reduced incidence of reoperation for repair failure (2). It is generally accepted that some sort of mechanical support is necessary to maintain the integrity of the repair, though some argue it can be used selectively (3,4). If some residual regurgitation is noted upon completion, the annuloplasty should prevent progression. Many different types of annuloplasty techniques have been described, some using plicating sutures, circumferential shortening sutures, bands to support the posterior annulus, and complete rings. Rings also have been rigid, semirigid, and completely flexible. Each technique has certain advantages and disadvantages. Rigid and semirigid rings enforce size reduction and shape change on the annulus, converting the native saddle-shaped annulus to a flat plane and restricting deformation through the cardiac cycle. Bands are designed to support the muscular annulus presuming that most of the change in annular size with regurgitation occurs there rather than in the fibrous anterior portion of the annulus. David examined a small group of patients (twenty-five) randomized to receive a rigid or flexible ring, and noted better systolic function in those with a flexible ring on short-term follow-up (5), though this was discounted by Carpentier as the differences disappeared on long-term follow-up (6). Unger-Graeber studied 122 patients who had repairs with a rigid or flexible ring or no ring and found that patients with rings have statistically significant, but clinically unimportant, reductions in valve area but no difference in diastolic velocity or gradient (7), while Detter et al. found similar results comparing a mural annulus shortening suture to a Carpentier-Edwards prosthetic ring (8). In contrast, Grossi et al. noted a survival benefit in patients with functional ischemic mitral regurgitation treated with ring annuloplasty in contrast to simple suture repair (9) and Czer et al. noted that ring annuloplasty was more effective in reducing and achieving a lower residual grade of regurgitation than commissural annuloplasty (10). Komoda et al. noted that a posterior pericardial annuloplasty tightly anchored to the trigones bilaterally eliminated breakdown after Gerbode plasty, in contrast to Paneth suture annuloplasty (11).

Good results have been reported with all annuloplasty techniques, perhaps the best approach is to choose a technique, learn it, and consistently apply it to maximize chances of consistent long-term success.

SUTURE ANNULOPLASTY

Commissural Annuloplasty

Reed described a commissural annuloplasty called a "measured mitral annuloplasty" in 1965 (Fig. 6.1) (12). In 1980 he published 17-year results, describing 196 patients treated from 1961 to 1978, 35% of patients had been operated on for isolated mitral valve disease, 115 had annuloplasty and 81 had commissurotomy and annuloplasty. The age range was from 3 to 70 years. Reoperation was required in 8.7% of the patients (13).

Posterior Annuloplasty

Kay Annuloplasty

Kay et al. described a posterior suture annuloplasty using figure-of-eight sutures to reduce the posterior annulus circumference by one third (14) (Fig. 6.2).

Gerbode Annuloplasty

Gerbode described a posterior folding plasty similar to the Kay annuloplasty but in the center of the posterior leaflet (15) (Fig. 6.3).

Komoda et al. reviewed their experience with this technique noting the results with simple Gerbode plasty, Gerbode plasty with Paneth annuloplasty, and Gerbode plasty with loose reinforcement with a pericardial strip produced inadequate results. The cause of failure was the breakdown of the plication by the Gerbode plasty; however, Gerbode plasty combined with a tightly anchored pericardial strip from trigone to trigone produced excellent results (11) (Fig. 6.4). Note this technique creates a functional unileaflet valve.

Paneth Annuloplasty

Burr et al. described a circumferential mitral plication suture (Paneth-Burr method) (Fig. 6.5) which consisted of two sutures forming a U anchored in the central fibrous body on each side and running respectively around the left and right sides of the annulus, as a parallel double layer, to the midpoint of the posterior leaflet, and tied over a pledget (16). Though good results were reported in early follow-up, in 80 patients with good follow-up, they noted early failures in 13 patients, 7 for progression of rheumatic disease. They recommended not using the technique in elderly patients with rheumatic disease (17). In a sheep

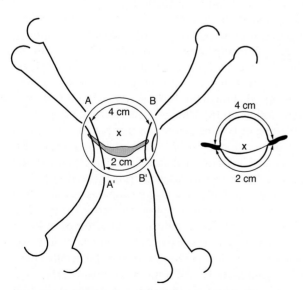

Figure 6.1   Commissural annuloplasty. (From Reed GE. Repair of mitral regurgitation. An 11-year experience. *Am J Cardiol.* 1973:31:494–496.)

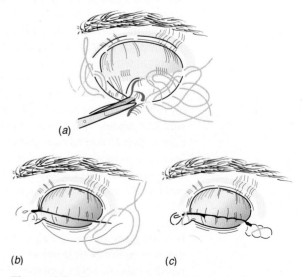

Figure 6.2   Kay posterior annuloplasty. (From Kay JH, Zubiate P, Mendez AM, Carpena C, Watanabe K, Magidson O. Mitral valve repair for patients with pure mitral insufficiency. 1- to 15-year follow-up. *JAMA.* 1976;236:1584–1586.)

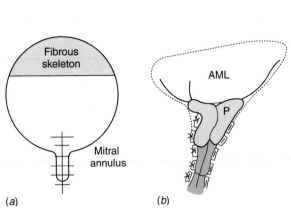

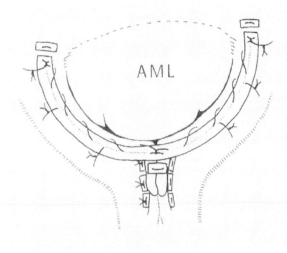

Figure 6.3 Gerbode Posterior Plasty; schematic (**A**); surgical appearance (**B**); AML, anterior mitral leaflet; P, posterior mitral leaflet. (From Komoda T, Hubler M, Siniawski H, Hetzer R. Annular stabilization in mitral repair without a prosthetic ring. *J Heart Valve Dis.* 2000;9:776–782.)

Figure 6.4 Gerbode plasty reinforced with a posterior pericardial strip. The strip is sewn to the annulus with approximating sutures then secured with a running suture. (From Komoda T, Hubler M, Siniawski H, Hetzer R. Annular stabilization in mitral repair without a prosthetic ring. *J Heart Valve Dis.* 2000;9:776–782.)

model, Tibayan et al. demonstrated that suture annuloplasty preserved annular and leaflet motion in contrast to the restriction of annular and leaflet motion by a ring (18).

Ricchi et al. describes a variation of this with one running suture line parallel to the annulus (Fig. 6.6) and the other placed perpendicular to the annulus in three segments around the posterior annulus to allow adjustment (Fig. 6.7) (19).

Barlow recently described using multiple annular sutures (Fig. 6.8) to create multiple plications of the annulus (20). This technique was used in 60 patients, over 124 months, with no failures after a mean follow-up of 29 months. They recommend use of an annuloplasty ring in the presence of gross annular degeneration or severe dilatation, if an optimal result has not been achieved without a ring, if the annulus requires extensive decalcification, or if the etiology is rheumatic or ischemic disease.

Suture Annuloplasty through the Ventricle

Menicanti et al. describe posterior suture annuloplasty through the left ventriculotomy as a component of the Dor procedure (21). As detailed in Fig. 6.9, the pledgeted 2-0 suture is

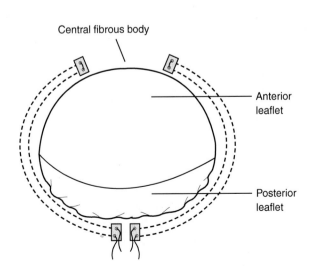

Figure 6.5 Paneth-Burr posterior suture annuloplasty. (From Burr LH, Krayenbuhl C, Sutton MSJ, Paneth M. The mitral plication suture. A new technique of mitral valve repair. *J Thorac Cardiovasc Surg.* 1977;73:589–595.)

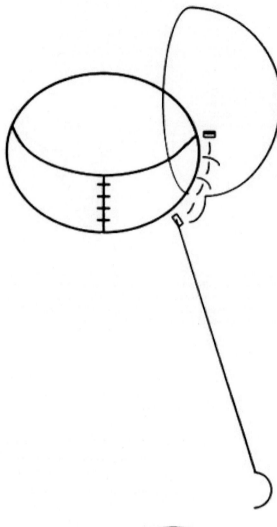

Figure 6.6 Linear segmental annuloplasty. The first segment of the posterior mitral annulus is encircled with 2/0 polypropylene suture. (From Ricchi A, Ortu P, Cirio EM, Falchi S, Lixi G, Martelli V. Linear segmental annuloplasty for mitral valve repair. *Ann Thorac Surg.* 1997;63:1805–1806.)

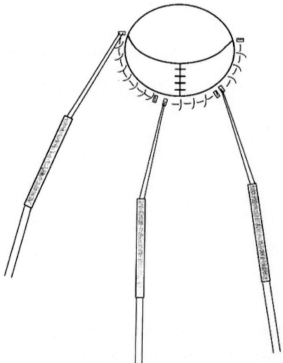

Figure 6.7 Linear segmental annuloplasty. The three 2/0 polypropylene sutures are passed in tourniquets. (From Ricchi A, Ortu P, Cirio EM, Falchi S, Lixi G, Martelli V. Linear segmental annuloplasty for mitral valve repair. *Ann Thorac Surg.* 1997;63:1805–1806.)

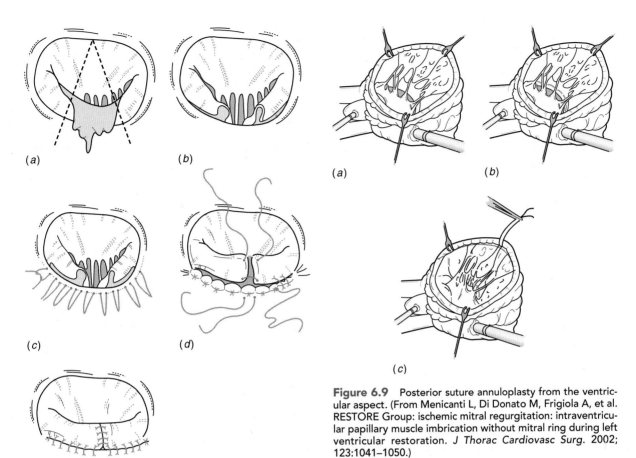

(a)   (b)

(c)   (d)

(e)

(a)   (b)

(c)

Figure 6.9   Posterior suture annuloplasty from the ventricular aspect. (From Menicanti L, Di Donato M, Frigiola A, et al. RESTORE Group: ischemic mitral regurgitation: intraventricular papillary muscle imbrication without mitral ring during left ventricular restoration. *J Thorac Cardiovasc Surg.* 2002; 123:1041–1050.)

Figure 6.8   Suture annuloplasty. (From Barlow CW, Ali ZA, Lim E, Barlow JB, Wells FC. Modified technique for mitral repair without ring annuloplasty. *Ann Thorac Surg.* 2003; 75:298–300.)

brought from the ventricular to the atrial side at the right trigone, run along the annulus then brought back through to the ventricular side at the left trigone and tied over a pledget. A 23-millimeter valve sizer is used to calibrate the orifice size while tying.

RING OR BAND ANNULOPLASTY

Overview of Available Annular Support Prostheses

Though there are differences of opinion, most surgeons agree that durability of the repair is enhanced by some sort of structural support. As discussed in Chapter 2, on anatomy, the annular support of the valve is the fibrous and muscular portion and the transition point is the fibrous trigones. The annular support performs a dual role: shrinking the dilated annulus, returning the mitral orifice area toward normal allowing coaptation of the leaflets and preventing recurrent dilation leading to failure of the repair. Rings completely encircle the annulus and bands support the posterior annulus from trigone to trigone; they can be adjustable, rigid, semirigid or flexible. Flexible rings and bands are usually attached to a template to support them and prevent crimping (which can lead to foreshortening of the circumference) while tying. A circumferential ring may be preferable for a large ventricle secondary to cardiomyopathy or chronic ischemic disease in which annuloplasty is the principle component of the repair (22–24).

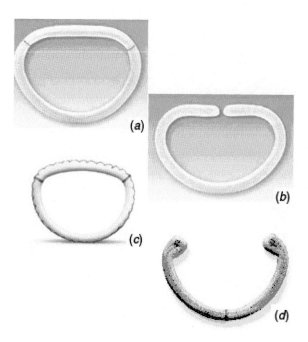

Figure 6.10   Rigid and semirigid rings and bands.

Rigid and Semirigid Rings

Among the first manufactured prostheses was a rigid ring designed by Carpentier (Fig. 6.10A). This ring was designed to have an anterior-posterior to side-to-side ratio of 3:4. Made of titanium and covered with a polyester knit, this ring encircles and immobilizes the annulus. Similar in design is a semirigid ring, which is manufactured in a similar shape and proportion; the portion that attaches to the muscular annulus is somewhat flexible but its deformity is limited (Fig. 6.10B,C). Sequin's semirigid ring is made with a flexible core that is high strength and fatigue resistant (Fig. 6.11) (25). Gradual reduction of the ring diameter increases flexibility around the posterior leaflet. This fixes the annulus and allows annular deformation. Resistance to longitudinal deformation prevents bunching while the ring is tied down. Semirigid bands are also available (Fig. 6.10D). New concepts for rigid and semirigid ring design are being explored; for example, an asymmetric ring for relatively greater reduction of the P3 segment for ischemia-induced regurgitation has recently been introduced.

Flexible Rings

Flexible rings and bands have no intrinsic shape and conform to the shape of the annulus tending to make it more circular instead of the D shape forced by a rigid ring (Fig. 6.12). Flexible prostheses will prevent radial expansion but not limit three-dimensional motion

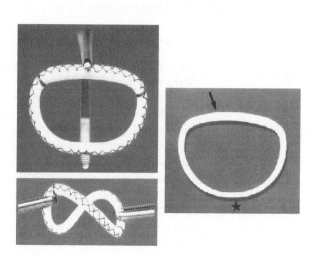

Figure 6.11   Seguin semirigid ring. (see text) (From Seguin JR, Demaria R, Chaptal PA. Preservation of three-dimensional annular movement with the SJM, seguin mitral annuloplasty ring. *J Heart Valve Dis.* 1996;5:641–646.)

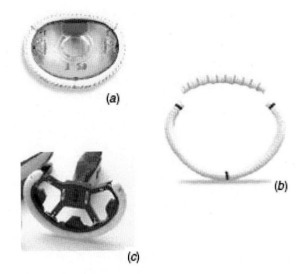

Figure 6.12 Complete and partial flexible rings and bands.

like a rigid or semirigid prosthesis does. The prosthesis is mounted on a tying template to prevent crimping during tying. The diameter of the mitral orifice can be adjusted during knot tying, depending on how much crimping is created. In addition, some flexible rings are designed to be adjustable, allowing the surgeon to shrink the circumference after tying the ring down, (Fig. 6.13), though Dr. A. Carpentier cautions against using an adjustable ring to compensate for an inadequate repair (personal communcation). Some flexible rings are designed to be used either as a ring or as a band, allowing a portion of the ring to be cut out as necessary (Fig. 6.12B).

A number of authors report success using other available materials to support repair. Chang et al. used a 3-millimeter wide strip of polytetrafluoroethylene (PTFE) graft material

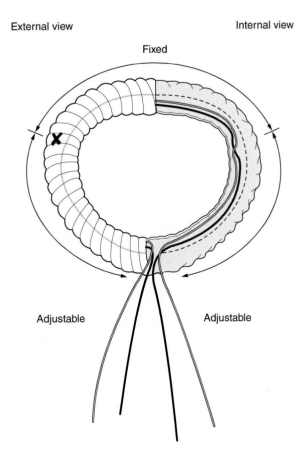

Figure 6.13 Adjustable flexible ring. (From Gorton ME, Piehler JM, Killen DA, Hoskins ML, Borkon AM. Mitral valve repair using a flexible and adjustable annuloplasty ring. *Ann Thorac Surg.* 1993;55:860–863.)

tailored to the length of the free edge of the anterior leaflet and sewn to the posterior annulus between the commissures (26). Others have reported the use of saphenous vein (27), autologous pericardium (28), and Dacron. Scrofani et al. reported good long-term results with gluteraldehyde-treated pericardium sewn in place from commissure to commissure with mattress sutures to create an orifice of two finger breadths (29). Though this is in contrast to results presented by Bevilacqua et al. who noted a five-year freedom from reoperation rate of 90.1% for the Carpentier-Edwards ring and 62.6% for a posterior pericardial band (30); most frequently from suture dehiscence of posterior annulus plication and leaflet reconstruction with partial ring detachment.

Which Band Should Be Used and When?

Though there are many different brands with minor differences between them, they all are either bands or rings, rigid or flexible, with a fixed or adjustable circumference. Usage depends on the surgeon; for most situations, any prosthesis will perform the primary role of support. However, some recommendations for use of specific prostheses in selected situations can be made. In general, a band will provide good support when the leaflet repair itself reduces annular circumference. A band is also useful if the anterior portion of the annulus is difficult to visualize. A complete ring may provide more support in a situation in which the surgeon relies on the ring to reduce annular circumference, for example a simple annuloplasty for ischemic disease or dilated cardiomyopathy. Rigid rings have been more prone to the creation of systolic anterior motion, however, techniques that restrict the height of the posterior leaflet prevent this. Okada et al. compared Carpentier and Duran rings noting greater left ventricular fractional shortening and lower peak velocity with the flexible Duran ring (31); the clinical significance of this is unclear. Most prostheses are not adjustable, however, Gorton et al. reported adjustment after attachment to reduce or eliminate residual regurgitation was beneficial in 9 of 21 patients (32). Borghetti et al. examined the relative effects of a rigid (Carpentier-Edwards) vs. flexible (autologous pericardium) annuloplasty ring (33). They noted only one major difference—improvement in the ejection fraction with exercise with the flexible ring, which they attributed to improved mitral annular systolic excursion. In contrast, Bevilacqua et al. noted inferior long-term results with glutaralehyde-treated autologous pericardial posterior annuloplasty in comparison to the standard Carpentier ring (34). Gillinov reported midterm results with the Cosgrove-Edwards annuloplasty band, describing at a mean follow-up interval of 18 months no MR or 1+ MR in 80% of patients (35), and stated that results with a posterior annuloplasty were equivalent to circumferential annuloplasty (36).

INSERTION TECHNIQUE

In general proper ring (band) insertion will require 13–25 (9–20) sutures depending on the degree of annular dilation. Sutures can be placed parallel or radial to the annulus. If parallel to the annulus, sutures should be placed at a depth of between 2 and 3 millimeters with a width of between 4 and 5 millimeters. For a very large annulus, consideration should be given to placing many narrowly placed sutures or overlapping sutures for additional security. Care must be taken to insert the sutures in the annular/atrial tissue and not the leaflet tissue; it is important not to impede the hinge function of the leaflet (A. Carpentier, personal communication). When placed through the ring, sutures from the fibrous portion of the annulus should be placed at a width similar to that of the annular suture because no annular reduction is anticipated for the fibrous portion. In contrast the width of the sutures for the posterior annulus is much smaller on the ring, facilitating size reduction. The approach is similar for radial sutures taking care to avoid gaps between the ring and the annulus. Care should be taken not to alter the circumference of the ring while tying. Rigid and semirigid rings will not deform. However, when tied, horizontal sutures will bunch up flexible rings. Tying sutures while the ring or band is attached to the template it is mounted on will prevent this. Often flexible rings and bands are mounted on a template that is not of the classic 3:4 proportion,

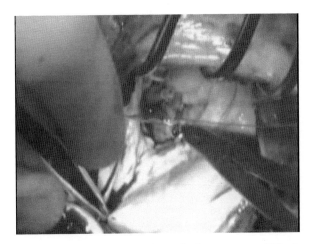

Figure 6.14 Placement of annuloplasty sutures. (Clip 4, Case 4)

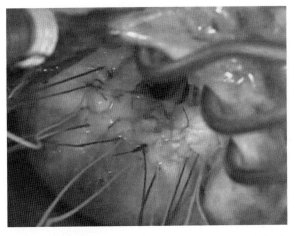

Figure 6.15 Placement of annuloplasty sutures. (Clip 8, Case 1)

but wider in the lateral dimension and narrower in the anterior-posterior dimension, requiring that the ring or band be cut off the template sequentially as it is sewn down; after a portion of sutures are tied while attached to the template to prevent crimping, the suture holding the prosthesis on the template is cut and the prosthesis avulsed off the template. Begin at the left trigone, tying 3 or 4 sutures, then cut the retention suture on the anterior annulus and avulse the left trigone area, proceeding around the right trigone and alternating on each side to the middle of the posterior annulus in a similar fashion. This allows the ring or band to be secured in place without crimping the prosthesis (Figs. 6.14–6.17).

SIZING

Ring sizing and placement may vary among manufacturers. As a general rule, the mitral annulus should have a surface area similar to that of the anterior leaflet. With a ring sized to a 3:4 ratio, the intertrigonal distance will be proportional to the anterior leaflet size and used to select a ring (A. Carpentier uses the intercommissural distance, personal communication). The central anterior-posterior diameter (height) of the anterior leaflet should equal that of the ring. Ideal sizing should reduce annular size to produce a surface of coaptive contact of at least 0.5 mm between the anterior and posterior leaflets. In situations of annular reduction for cardiomyopathy and ischemic disease some surgeons advocate placing the smallest ring possible. Though it is theoretically possible to create mitral stenosis, significant stenosis is unusual with simple annular reduction (Figs. 6.18–6.22).

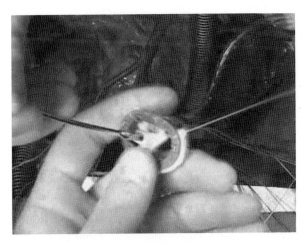

Figure 6.16 Placement of sutures through the annuloplasty band. (Clip 10, Case 1)

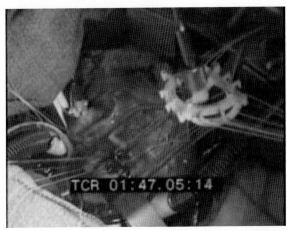

Figure 6.17 Securing the ring. (Clip 8, Case 6)

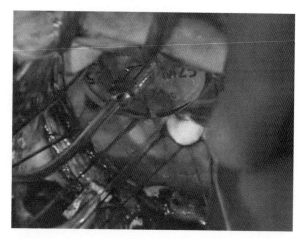

Figure 6.18   Sizing the annuloplasty ring. (Clip 4, Case 2)

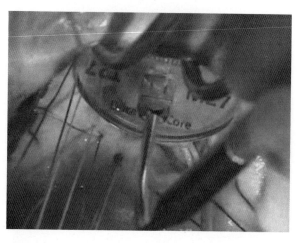

Figure 6.19   Sizing the annuloplasty band. (Clip 5, Case 3)

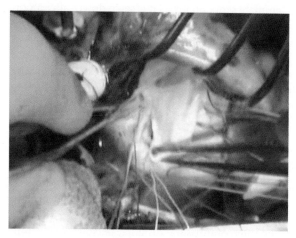

Figure 6.20   Sizing the annuloplasty band. (Clip 5, Case 4)

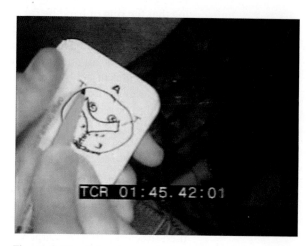

Figure 6.21   Sizing the annuloplasty ring. (Clip 7, Case 6)

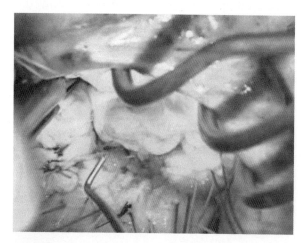

Figure 6.22   Sizing the annuloplasty band. (Clip 9, Case 1)

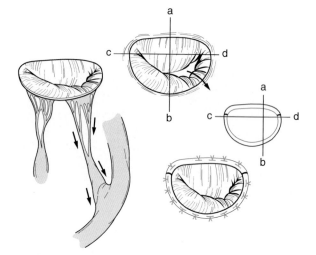

Figure 6.23   Asymmetric annuloplasty. (From Chitwood Jr. WR. Mitral valve repair: ischemic. In: Kaiser LR, Kron IL, Spray TL. *Mastery of Cardiothoracic Surgery*. Philadelphia: Lippincott-Raven, 1998:317.)

Asymmetric Annuloplasty

Various techniques exist to deal with the asymmetry of ischemic mitral regurgitation. One of these techniques is asymmetric placement of the annuloplasty ring to compensate for the asymmetry of the posterior leaflet abnormality (37). This technique is demonstrated in (Fig. 6.23). Note a greater reduction in the annular circumference between points b and d relative to that between b and c. As stated above newer rings have been designed to replicate this approach.

REFERENCES

1. Scrofani R, Santoli C. The role of annuloplasty in mitral valve repair. *J Thorac Cardiovasc Surg.* 1997;113:957–958.
2. Cohn LH, Couper GS, Aranki SF, Rizzo RJ, Kinchla NM, Collins JJ Jr. Long-term results of mitral valve reconstruction for regurgitation of the myxomatous mitral valve. *J Thorac Cardiovasc Surg.* 1994;107:143–150.
3. Milano A, Codecasa R, DeCarlo M, et al. Mitral valve annuloplasty for degenerative disease: assessment of four different techniques. *J Heart Valve Dis.* 2000;9:321–326.
4. Alvarez JM, Deal CW, Loveridge K. Repairing the degenerative mitral valve: ten- to fifteen-year follow-up. *J Thorac Cardiovasc Surg.* 1996;112:238–247.
5. David TE, Komeda M, Pollick C, Burns RJ. Mitral valve annuloplasty: the effect of the type on left ventricular function. *Ann Thorac Surg.* 1989;47:524–527.
6. Carpentier A. Mitral valve annuloplasty. *Ann Thorac Surg.* 1990;49:508–509.
7. Unger-Graeber B, Lee RT, Sutton MS, et al. Doppler echocardiographic comparison of the Carpentier and Duran annuloplasty rings versus no ring after mitral valve repair for mitral regurgitation. *Am J Cardiol.* 1991;67:517–519.
8. Detter C, Aybek T, Kupilik N, Fischlein T, Moritz A. Mitral valve annuloplasty: comparison of the mural annulus shortening suture (MASS) with the Carpentier-Edwards prosthetic ring. *J Heart Valve Dis.* 2000;9:478–486.
9. Grossi EA, Bizekis CS, LaPietra A, et al. Late results of isolated mitral annuloplasty for "functional" ischemic mitral insufficiency. *J Card Surg.* 2001;16:328–332.
10. Czer LS, Maurer G, Trento A, et al. Comparative efficacy of ring and suture annuloplasty for ischemic mitral regurgitation. *Circulation.* 1992;86:II46–52.
11. Komoda T, Hubler M, Siniawski H, Hetzer R. Annular stabilization in mitral repair without a prosthetic ring. *J Heart Valve Dis.* 2000;9:776–782.
12. Reed GE, Tice DA, Clauss RH. Asymmetric exaggerated mitral annuloplasty: repair of mitral insufficiency with hemodynamic predictability. *J Thorac Cardiovasc Surg.* 1965;49:752.
13. Reed GE, Pooley RW, Moggio RA: Durability of measured mitral annuloplasty; 17 year study. *J Thorac Cardiovasc Surg.* 1980;79:321.
14. Kay JH, Zubiate P, Mendez AM, Carpena C, Watanabe K, Magidson O. Mitral valve repair for patients with pure mitral insufficiency. 1- to 15-year follow-up. *JAMA.* 1976;236:1584–1586.
15. Gerbode F, Kerth WJ, Osborn JJ, Selzer A. Correction of mitral insufficiency by open operation. *Ann Surg.* 1962;155:846–854.
16. Burr LH, Krayenbuhl C, Sutton MSJ, Paneth M. The mitral plication suture. A new technique of mitral valve repair. *J Thorac Cardiovasc Surg.* 1977;73:589–595.
17. Shore DF, Wong P, Paneth M: Results of mitral valvuloplasty with a suture plication technique. *J Thorac Cardiovasc Surg* 1980;79:349–357.
18. Tibayan FA, Rodriguez F, Liang D, Daughters GT, Ingels NB Jr, Miller DC. Paneth suture annuloplasty abolishes acute ischemic mitral regurgitation but preserves annular and leaflet dynamics. *Circulation.* 2003;108 Suppl 1:II128–33.
19. Ricchi A, Ortu P, Cirio EM, Falchi S, Lixi G, Martelli V. Linear segmental annuloplasty for mitral valve repair. *Ann Thorac Surg.* 1997;63:1805–1806.
20. Barlow CW, Ali ZA, Lim E, Barlow JB, Wells FC. Modified technique for mitral repair without ring annuloplasty. *Ann Thorac Surg.* 2003;75:298–300.
21. Menicanti L, Di Donato M, Frigiola A, et al. RESTORE Group: ischemic mitral regurgitation: intraventricular papillary muscle imbrication without mitral ring during left ventricular restoration. *J Thorac Cardiovasc Surg.* 2002;123:1041–1050.
22. Sanders JH Jr, Scott ML. Pitfalls in surgical decision-making during mitral valve repair. *Curr Opin Cardiol.* 2001;16:140–145.
23. Gorman JH 3rd, Gorman RC, Jackson BM, Enomoto Y, St John-Sutton MG, Edmunds LH Jr. Annuloplasty ring selection for chronic ischemic mitral regurgitation: lessons from the ovine model. *Ann Thorac Surg.* 2003;76:1556–1563.
24. Tibayan FA, Rodriguez F, Langer F. Annular remodeling in chronic ischemic mitral regurgitation: ring selection implications. *Ann Thorac Surg.* 2003;76:1549–1554.
25. Seguin JR, Demaria R, Chaptal PA. Preservation of three-dimensional annular movement with the SJM-Seguin mitral annuloplasty ring. *J Heart Valve Dis.* 1996;5:641–646.
26. Chang CH, Lin PJ, Chang JP, Chu JJ, Hsieh MJ, Chiang CW. Long-term results of polytetrafluoroethylene mitral annuloplasty. *Ann Thorac Surg.* 1994;57:644–647.
27. Paruchuru PK, Adluri K, Alzetani A, Patel R. Mitral annuloplasty with autologous pericardium and saphenous vein. *Asian Cardiovasc Thorac Ann.* 2003;11:83–84.
28. Salvador L, Rocco F, Ius P, et al. The pericardium reinforced suture annuloplasty: another tool available for mitral annulus repair? *J Card Surg.* 1993;8:79–84.
29. Scrofani R, Moriggia S, Salati M, Fundaro P, Danna P, Santoli C. Mitral valve remodeling: long-term results with posterior pericardial annuloplasty. *Ann Thorac Surg.* 1996;61:895–899.
30. Bevilacqua S, Cerillo AG, Gianetti J, et al. Mitral valve repair for degenerative disease: is pericardial posterior annuloplasty a durable option? *Eur J Cardiothorac Surg.* 2003;23:552–559.
31. Okada Y, Shomura T, Yamaura Y, Yoshikawa J. Comparison of the Carpentier and Duran prosthetic rings used in mitral reconstruction. *Ann Thorac Surg.* 1995;59:658–662.
32. Gorton ME, Peihler JM, Killen DA, Hoskins ML, Borkon AM. Mitral valve repair using a flexible and adjustable annuloplasty ring. *Ann Thorac Surg.* 1993;55:860–863.
33. Borghetti V, Campana M, Scotti C, et al. Biological versus prosthetic ring in mitral-valve repair: enhancement of mitral annulus dynamics and left-ventricular function with pericardial annuloplasty at long term. *Eur J Cardiothorac Surg.* 2000;17:431–439.
34. Bevilacqua S, Cerillo AG, Gianetti J, et al. Mitral valve repair for degenerative disease: is pericardial posterior annuloplasty a durable option? *Eur J Cardiothorac Surg.* 2003;23:552–559.
35. Gillinov AM, Cosgrove DM 3rd, Shiota T, Qin J, et al. Cosgrove-Edwards annuloplasty system: midterm results. *Ann Thorac Surg.* 2000;69:717–721.
36. Gillinov AM, Cosgrove DM. Mitral valve repair for degenerative disease. *J Heart Valve Dis.* 2002;11 Suppl 1:S15–20.
37. David T. Techniques and results of mitral valve repair for ischemic mitral regurgitation. *J Card Surg.* 1994;9:274.

Commissurotomy

7

There is a continued role for open mitral commissurotomy for valves that remain pliable despite rheumatic changes. The technique involves sharply dividing the fused leaflets (Fig. 7.1) and separating the fused chordae (Fig. 7.2) to the anterior and posterior leaflets (Fig. 7.3). Great care should be taken to insure that the valve is competent on closure and pliable enough to open with minimal pressure.

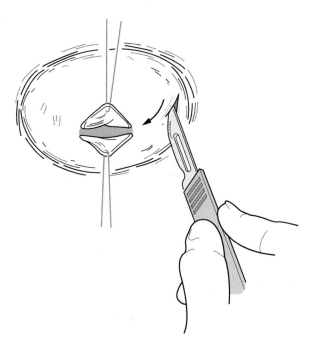

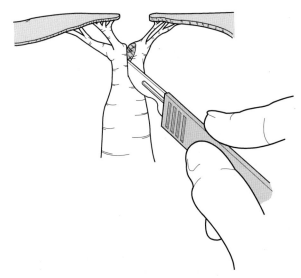

Figure 7.1 Commissural division. After the placement of stay sutures the commissure is carefully divided with a scalpel along the line of fusion next to, but not extending to, the annulus. (From Kouchoukos NT, Blackstone EH, Doty DB, Hanley FL, Karp RB. Kirklin/Barratt-Boyes cardiac surgery: morphology, diagnostic criteria, natural history, techniques, results, and indications. Philadelphia: Churchill Livingstone; 2003: 493.)

Figure 7.2 Lysis of fused chordae. (From Kouchoukos NT, Blackstone EH, Doty DB, Hanley FL, Karp RB. Kirklin/Barratt-Boyes cardiac surgery: morphology, diagnostic criteria, natural history, techniques, results, and indications. Philadelphia: Churchill Livingstone; 2003:493.)

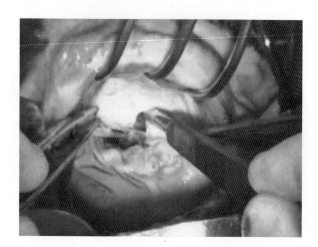

Figure 7.3   Commissurotomy (Clip 4, Case 3)

Anterior Leaflet
Repair Techniques

8

Unlike the posterior leaflet, which has broad annular attachment and can be immobilized and forced to act as an abutment for the functioning anterior leaflet, the anterior leaflet has narrow annular attachment and a broad occlusive surface area that must function properly for mitral competency. Therefore, repair of the anterior leaflet requires more imagination, often requires a combination of repair techniques, and is considered more prone to failure on long-term follow-up. However, this assumption is contraindicated by Grossi et al. who found, after reviewing 588 consecutive repairs, that the requirement for anterior leaflet repair did not increase the risk for reoperation (1).

General principles of anterior leaflet repair include elimination of redundancy and excess tissue, elimination of prolapse, and maintenance of pliability. The leaflet's motion must allow adequate diastolic flow avoiding stenosis yet adequately occlude the mitral orifice during systole, eliminating regurgitation. Leaflet interventions must be durable and resistant to functional alterations related to healing.

This chapter will deal specifically with techniques used to alter the leaflet shape and size; chordal repair techniques are detailed in Chapter 11.

TRIANGULAR RESECTION

Early in the history of valve repair concern was expressed regarding the longevity of anterior triangular resection (2), however, Grossi et al. reported excellent results and advocate appropriate application of this procedure (1,3). Separately described recently by Fasol (4) (Fig. 8.1) and Spencer et al. (5), the technique involves the resection of a narrow isosceles triangle of tissue, excising no more than 1.5 cm of prolapsing leaflet tissue. The excision is made to a strong chord on each side. Spencer et al. (5) routinely apply this technique for focal anterior leaflet prolapse, preferring it to shortening or transferring chords.

Most recently Fasol and Mahdjoobian described a combined anterior triangular resection and posterior quadrangular resection with folding plasty (see Chapter 9) for Barlow's disease with good short-term results in 37 patients (Fig. 8.2) (6).

LEAFLET SHORTENING

Shortening of the anterior leaflet by excision of an ellipse of tissue (elliptoid excision) has been described (7), however no series detailing the success of this technique were found. A refined description of this technique was made by Duran (8) (Fig. 8.3). The upper incision is made 5 mm from the annulus. Tissue is removed to create a final leaflet height of

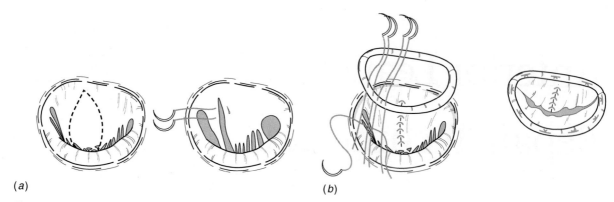

(a)   *(b)*

Figure 8.1   Anterior triangular resection. (From Fasol R, Joubert-Hubner E. Triangular resection of the anterior leaflet for repair of the mitral valve. *Ann Thorac Surg.* 2001; 71:381–383.)

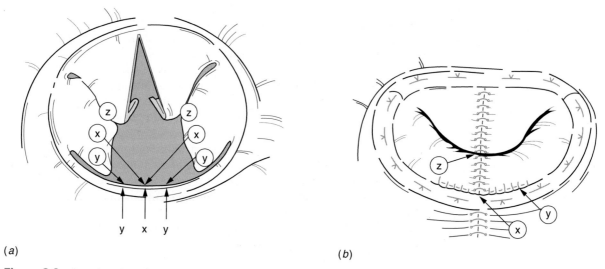

(a)   *(b)*

Figure 8.2   Anterior triangular resection and posterior quadrangular resection and folding plasty for Barlow's disease. (From Fasol R, Mahdjoobian K. Repair of mitral valve billowing and prolapse (Barlow): the surgical technique. *Ann Thorac Surg.* 2002;74:602–605.)

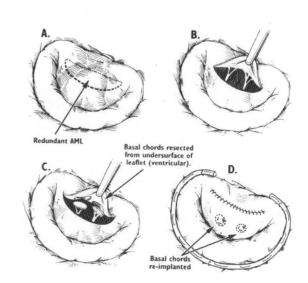

Figure 8.3   Anterior leaflet shortening. (From Duran CMG. Surgical techniques for the repair of anterior mitral leaflet prolapse. *J Card Surg.* 1999;14;471–481.)

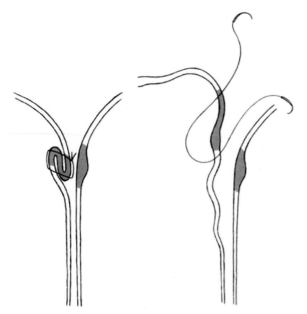

Figure 8.4 Technique of free edge remodeling. (From Fundaro P, Moneta A, Villa E, et al. Chordal plication and free edge remodeling for mitral anterior leaflet prolapse repair: 8-year follow-up. *Ann Thorac Surg.* 2001;72:1515–1519.)

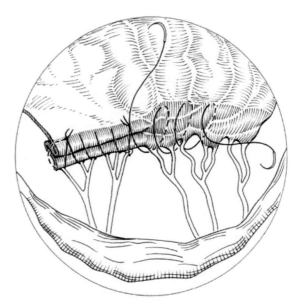

Figure 8.5 Technique of free edge remodeling. (From Fundaro P, Moneta A, Villa E, et al. Chordal plication and free edge remodeling for mitral anterior leaflet prolapse repair: 8-year follow-up. *Ann Thorac Surg.* 2001;72:1515–1519.)

between 25 and 30 mm. Major basal chords attached to the removed leaflet tissue are repositioned to maintain ventricular function. The use of this procedure to correct SAM (systolic anterior motion) was reported by Raney et al. who called it the Pomeroy Procedure (9).

FREE EDGE REMODELING

Demonstrated in Figures 8.4 and 8.5 are techniques described by Fundaro et al. as chordal suture plication and free edge remodeling (10). Reviewing 61 patients, they noted postoperative mitral regurgitation fell to 0.4 ± 0.7 from 3.7 ± 0.4. With mean follow-up of 40.5 months he reported 3 late deaths and 3 reoperations and actuarial overall survival, freedom from cardiac death, and freedom from mitral reoperation at 92 months of 85.1% ± 7.9%, 88.9% ± 7.7%, and 94.6% ± 3.0%. This technique can be used for focal or extensive prolapse. It is particularly useful for a focal area of prolapse or thickening on the anterior leaflet that prevents occlusive coaptation. The edge is pulled under to present a smooth portion of the anterior leaflet for apposition against the posterior leaflet.

OTHER METHODS TO DEAL WITH LEAFLET PROLAPSE

See Chapter 12.

LEAFLET AUGMENTATION

See Chapter 12.

REFERENCES

1. Grossi EA, Galloway AC, LaBoutillier M 3rd, et al. Anterior leaflet procedures during mitral valve repair do not adversely influence long-term outcome. *J Am Coll Cardiol.* 1995; 25:134–136.
2. Fucci C, Sandrelli L, Pardini A, Torracca L, Ferrari M, Alfieri O. Improved results with mitral valve repair using new surgical techniques. *Eur J Cardiothorac Surg.* 1995;9:621–626.

3. Grossi EA, LaPietra A, Galloway AC, Colvin SB. History of mitral valve anterior leaflet repair with triangular resection. *Ann Thorac Surg.* 2001;72:1794–1795.

4. Fasol R, Joubert-Hubner E. Triangular resection of the anterior leaflet for repair of the mitral valve. *Ann Thorac Surg.* 2001;71:381–383.

5. Spencer FC, Galloway AC, Grossi EA, et al. Recent developments and evolving techniques of mitral valve reconstruction. *Ann Thorac Surg.* 1998;65:307–313.

6. Fasol R, Mahdjoobian K. Repair of mitral valve billowing and prolapse (Barlow): the surgical technique. *Ann Thorac Surg.* 2002;74:602–605.

7. Quigley RL, Stagle RD. Alternative approach to the repair of a floppy anterior mitral valve leaflet. *J Heart Valve Dis.* 1995;4:208–210.

8. Duran CMG. Surgical techniques for the repair of anterior mitral leaflet prolapse. *J Card Surg.* 1999;14:471–481.

9. Raney AA, Shah PM, Joyo CI. The "Pomeroy procedure": a new method to correct post-mitral valve repair systolic anterior motion. *J Heart Valve Dis.* 2001;10:307–311.

10. Fundaro P, Moneta A, Villa E, et al. Chordal plication and free edge remodeling for mitral anterior leaflet prolapse repair: 8-year follow-up. *Ann Thorac Surg.* 2001;72:1515–1519.

Posterior Leaflet
Repair Techniques

9

POSTERIOR LEAFLET PLICATION

As the leaflets degenerate and become stiff and redundant with no clear major abnormalities that can be identified, the source of the leak may be attributable to incomplete closure of posterior leaflet clefts. This can result from redundancy or stiffness. A solution is to close the cleft by simple plication to reestablish the coaptive surface of the posterior leaflet (Figs. 9.1–9.3). This technique can also be used to exclude a prolapsing scallop or treat a posterior chordal rupture (1) (Fig. 9.4).

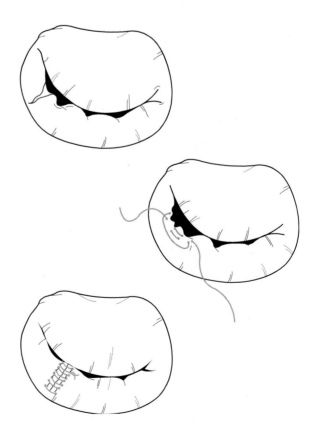

Figure 9.1 Posterior leaflet plication. (From Seccombe JF, Schaff HV. Mitral valve repair: current techniques and indications. In: Franco KL, Verrier ED, eds.: *Advanced Therapy in Cardiac Surgery*. St. Louis: B.C. Decker, 1999:224.)

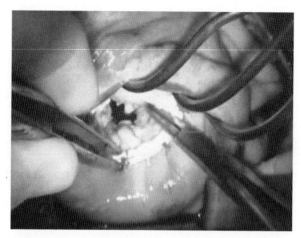

Figure 9.2 Cleft closure and lateral commissuroplasty. (Clip 6, Case 3)

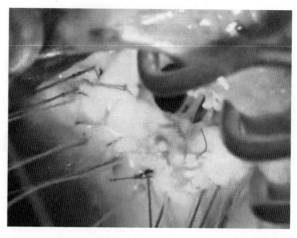

Figure 9.3 Cleft closure after posterior sliding plasty. (Clip 7, Case 1)

QUADRANGULAR RESECTION

One of the simplest and most commonly applied resection approaches is a quadrangular resection. The prolapsing portion of the leaflet is excised as a quadrangle to the annular level. The incision should be made in hardy tissue that will hold sutures well. The leaflets are then reapproximated with a running suture between the leaflet edges continuing to fold together the annular cut edges. The atrial portion can be reinforced with a pledgeted suture (Fig. 9.5). Suturing is started at the leaflet edge with a simple suture tied on the ventricular side of the valve that is brought through to the atrial side to pull the edge under (Fig. 9.6).

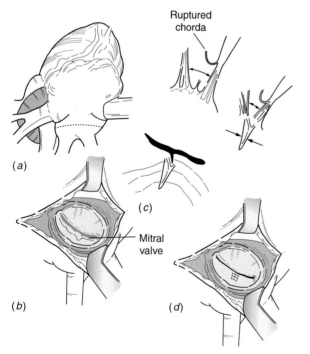

Figure 9.4 Posterior plication to treat a ruptured chord. **C:** View of the underside of the leaflet. (From McGoon DC. An early approach to the repair of ruptured mitral chordae. *Ann Thorac Surg.* 1989;47:628–629.)

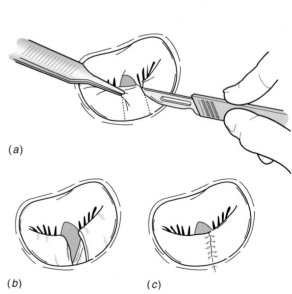

Figure 9.5 Quadrangular resection.

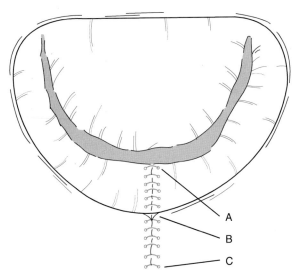

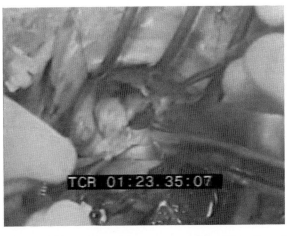

Figure 9.7 Quadrangular resection of the P2 scallop of the posterior leaflet. (Clip 2, Case 6)

Figure 9.6 Suture technique for quadrangular resection. The first of two layers is shown. **A:** Suture placed at the edge of the leaflets. **B:** Suture placed at the base of the annular plication. **C:** Suture placed at the apex of the annular plication.

This is then run as two layers in a running locking fashion (Fig. 5.6), reapproximating the cut edges of the leaflet taking care not to bunch up and foreshorten the leaflet. A second suture at the annulus pulls together the two cut edges at the annular level and the first suture is tied to this second, completing the leaflet reapproximation. This is then run to the apex of the annular fold and tied to a third anchoring suture. Completion of this repair may pull open a previously occlusive cleft between scallops, requiring simple closure with a figure-of-eight suture.

An alternative to excising the leaflet scallop is to fold down and plicate the redundant tissue. This is useful when the tissue is weak because there is more tissue to hold sutures in place (Figs. 9.7 and 9.8).

TRIANGULAR RESECTION

Seccombe and Schaff described a preference for triangular resection of the posterior leaflet for prolapse and redundancy of a large portion of the posterior leaflet (2). They felt this method placed less stress on the suture line and created less annular distortion (Fig. 9.9).

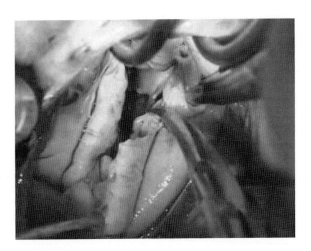

Figure 9.8 Excision of the P2 scallop based on the location of intact chords. (Clip 3, Case 1)

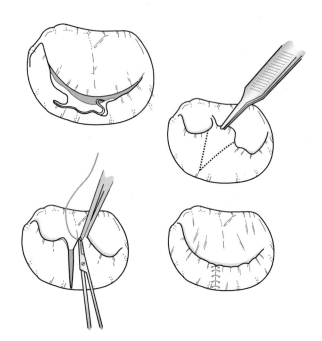

Figure 9.9 Posterior triangular resection. (From Seccombe JF, Schaff HV. Mitral valve repair: current techniques and indications. In: Franco KL, Verrier ED, eds. *Advanced Therapy in Cardiac Surgery*. St. Louis: B.C. Decker, 1999:225.)

SLIDING LEAFLET PLASTY

If the height of the posterior leaflet after quadrangular resection is too high (> 20 mm), there is an incidence of left ventricular outflow tract obstruction secondary to systolic anterior motion (See Chapter 12). To avoid this complication, Carpentier developed the sliding leaflet technique to remove excess tissue and preserve geometry (3). Perier et al. evaluated this technique in 48 patients with excellent results and no systolic anterior motion (SAM) (4).

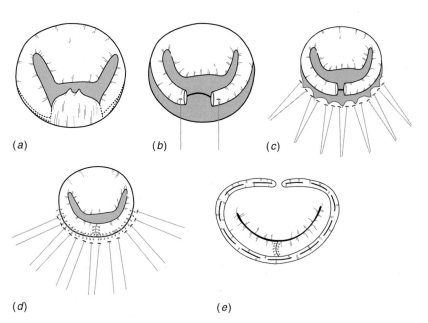

Figure 9.10 Sliding leaflet technique. (From Perier P, Clausnizer B, Mistarz K. Carpentier "sliding leaflet" technique for repair of the mitral valve: early results. *Ann Thorac Surg.* 1994;57:383–386.) **A:** A quadrangular resection of the diseased scallop is performed. **B:** The remaining posterior leaflet is detached from the annulus. **C:** Sutures are passed through the posterior annulus in a parallel orientation; the free edges of the leaflets are reapproximated. **D:** The leaflet is sewn to the annulus with a 4-0 monofilament and the leaflets reapproximated with 5-0 monofilament. **E:** The ring is secured in place.

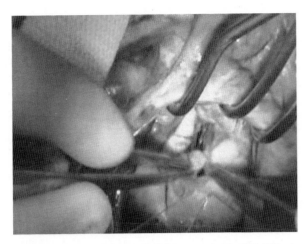

Figure 9.11 Mobilization of the posterior leaflet. (Clip 4, Case 1)

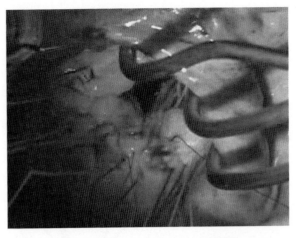

Figure 9.12 Reattachment of posterior leaflet creating a posterior sliding plasty. (Clip 5, Case 1)

Gillinov et al. recommend this technique be used instead of plication if the posterior leaflet excised is more than 1.5 centimeters (5) (Figs. 9.10–9.12).

A variant of this technique is described by Gillinov and Cosgrove for asymmetric leaflets in which one side is taller than the other because the quadrangular resection leaves leaflets of varying heights (6) (Figs. 9.13 and 9.14).

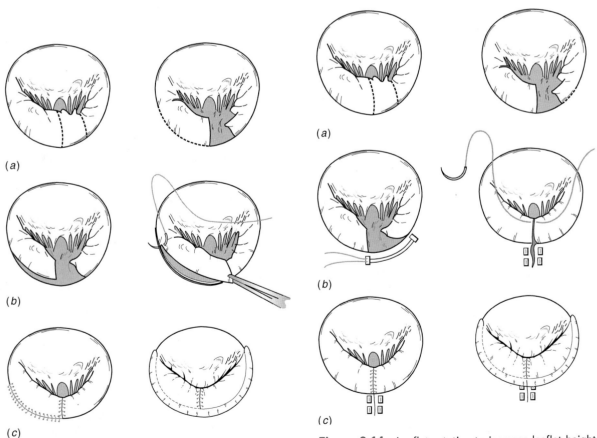

Figure 9.13 Modified sliding leaflet repair. (From Gillinov AM, Cosgrove DM. Modified quadrangular resection for mitral valve repair. *Ann Thorac Surg.* 2001;72:2153–2154.)

Figure 9.14 Leaflet rotation to increase leaflet height. (From Gillinov AM, Cosgrove DM. Modified quadrangular resection for mitral valve repair. *Ann Thorac Surg.* 2001; 72:2153–2154.)

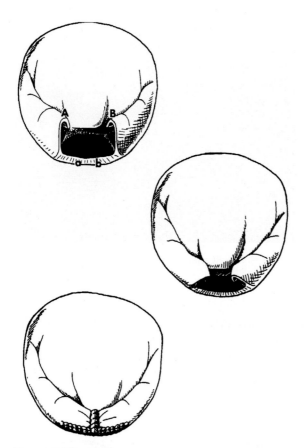

Figure 9.16   Posterior folding plasty. (Clip 4, Case 7)

Figure 9.15   Posterior folding plasty. (From Spencer FC, Galloway AC, Grossi EA, et al. Recent developments and evolving techniques of mitral valve reconstruction. *Ann Thorac Surg.* 1998;65:307–313.)

POSTERIOR FOLDING PLASTY

Another approach for a large redundant posterior leaflet is the posterior folding plasty described by Spencer et al. (7) (Figs. 9.15 and 9.16). Raman et al. described a variant of this procedure, which they called the double-breasted repair, and reported its application in 36 patients (8). In comparing this with standard quadrangular resection using annular plication they noted lower transmitral gradients (Fig. 9.17).

LEAFLET AUGMENTATION OR ADVANCEMENT

(See Chapter 11.)

REMOVAL OF ANNULAR CALCIFICATION

Debridement and Primary Closure

Described in 12 patients in 1991, debridement and primary closure involves extensive resection of the calcium with reconstruction of the annulus, using established methods of repair (9). This experience was updated by Carpentier et al. in 1996 (10). Reviewing 68 patients, they noted the calcification process was localized to the annu-

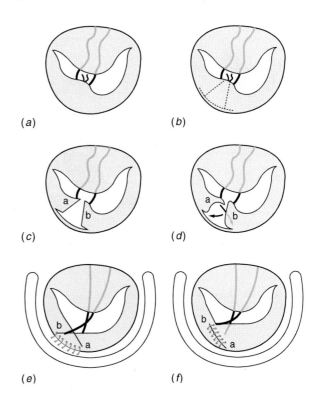

Figure 9.17 Double-breasted mitral valve repair. (From Raman JS, Gupta R, Shah P, Setty R, Tambara K. Double-breasted repair of the posterior mitral valve leaflet. *Ann Thorac Surg.* 2002;74:2206–2207.)

lus in 77% but could extend to the underlying myocardium. They fixed the valve by detaching of the leaflets, en bloc resection of the calcium deposit, annular reconstruction, and valve repair. If the calcification extended into the myocardium a sliding atrioplasty of the left atrium was performed. Actuarial freedom from reoperation was 87% at 7 years. They describe four differing degrees of calcification in the ventricle and leaflet (Fig. 9.18) in addition to various distribution patterns around the annulus. First the posterior leaflet is detached and the calcium removed by sharp dissection (Fig. 9.19). The annular defect is then closed with figure-of-eight 2-0 vertical sutures (Fig. 9.20). Stressing that "the ventricular bites of these sutures should involve only one third of the thickness of the myocardial wall and be as wide as possible, taking advantage of any fibrous tissue present on the surface of the endothelium."

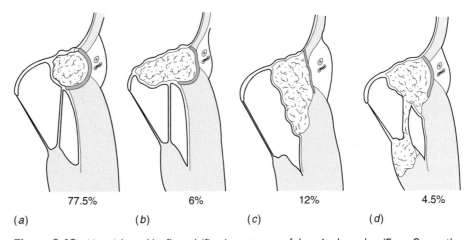

Figure 9.18 Ventricle and leaflet calcification patterns of the mitral annulus. (From Carpentier AF, Pellerin M, Fuzellier J, Relland JYM. Extensive calcification of the mitral valve annulus: pathology and surgical management. *J Thorac Cardiovasc Surg.* 1996;111:718–730.)

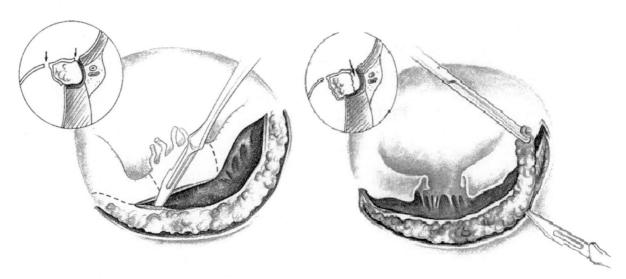

Figure 9.19 Annular decalcification. (From Carpentier AF, Pellerin M, Fuzellier J, Relland JYM. Extensive calcification of the mitral valve annulus: pathology and surgical management. *J Thorac Cardiovasc Surg.* 1996;111:718–730.)

If the defect extends far down into the myocardium he advocates the sliding atrium technique to repair it (Fig. 9.21). This technique moves the atrial wall into the ventricle to cover the defect and relocates the valve attachment point onto the atrial wall.

The leaflets are then reattached and an annuloplasty ring is placed with the sutures close to the annular defect (Fig. 9.22).

Debridement and Pericardial Patch Closure

David et al. described a similar approach to the one described above, patching the defect with pericardium instead of using primary repair (11) (Fig. 9.23). He also applied this technique for annular destruction by endocarditis.

Using a combination of these techniques in 37 patients, Ng et al. reported 1- and 5-year freedom of reoperation rates of 94.6% (12). Thirty-three had no to trivial regurgitation, and 3 had grade I–II regurgitation at follow-up. Similar results have been reported by other authors (13,14).

Figure 9.20 Repair of annular defect with vertical 2-0 figure-of-eight sutures. (From Carpentier AF, Pellerin M, Fuzellier J, Relland JYM. Extensive calcification of the mitral valve annulus: pathology and surgical management. *J Thorac Cardiovasc Surg.* 1996;111:718–730.)

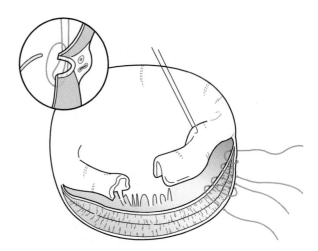

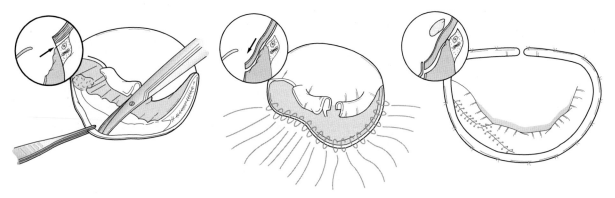

Figure 9.21 Sliding atrium technique. (From Carpentier AF, Pellerin M, Fuzellier J, Relland JYM. Extensive calcification of the mitral valve annulus: pathology and surgical management. *J Thorac Cardiovasc Surg.* 1996:111:718–730.)

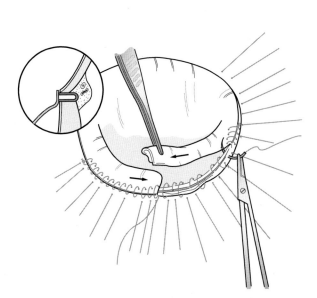

Figure 9.22 Reattaching the posterior leaflet. (From Carpentier AF, Pellerin M, Fuzellier J, Relland JYM. Extensive calcification of the mitral valve annulus: pathology and surgical management. *J Thorac Cardiovasc Surg.* 1996;111: 718–730.)

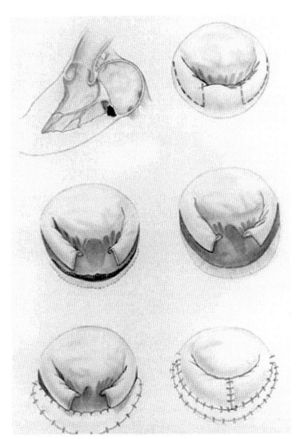

Figure 9.23 Annular reconstruction with pericardial patch. (From David TE, Feindel CM, Armstrong S, Sun Z. Reconstruction of the mitral annulus. A ten-year experience. *J Thorac Cardiovasc Surg.* 1995;110(5):1323–1332.)

REFERENCES

1. McGoon DC. An early approach to the repair of ruptured mitral chordae. *Ann Thorac Surg.* 1989;47:628–629.
2. Seccombe JF, Schaff HV. Mitral valve repair: current techniques and indications. In: Franco KL, Verrier ED, eds. *Advanced Therapy in Cardiac Surgery.* St. Louis: B.C. Decker. 1999:220–231.
3. Carpentier A. The sliding leaflet technique. *Le Club Mitrale Newsletter* 1998;I–5.
4. Perier P, Clausnizer B, Mistarz K. Carpentier "sliding leaflet" technique for repair of the mitral valve: early results. *Ann Thorac Surg.* 1994;57:383–386.
5. Gillinov AM, Cosgrove DM. Mitral valve repair for degenerative disease. *J Heart Valve Dis.* 2002;11 Suppl 1:S15–20.
6. Gillinov AM, Cosgrove DM. Modified quadrangular resection for mitral valve repair. *Ann Thorac Surg.* 2001;72:2153–2154.
7. Spencer FC, Galloway AC, Grossi EA, et al. Recent developments and evolving techniques of mitral valve reconstruction. *Ann Thorac Surg.* 1998;65:307–313.
8. Raman JS, Gupta R, Shah P, Setty R, Tambara K. Double-breasted repair of the posterior mitral valve leaflet. *Ann Thorac Surg.* 2002;74:2206–2207.
9. el Asmar B, Acker M, Couetil JP, et al. Mitral valve repair in the extensively calcified mitral valve annulus. *Ann Thorac Surg.* 1991;52:66–69.
10. Carpentier AF, Pellerin M, Fuzellier J, Relland JYM. Extensive calcification of the mitral valve annulus: pathology and surgical management. *J Thorac Cardiovasc Surg.* 1996;111:718–730.
11. David TE, Feindel CM, Armstrong S, Sun Z. Reconstruction of the mitral annulus. A ten-year experience. *J Thorac Cardiovasc Surg.* 1995;110(5):1323–1332.
12. Ng CK, Punzengruber C, Pachinger O, et al. Valve repair in mitral regurgitation complicated by severe annulus calcification. *Ann Thorac Surg.* 2000;70:53–58.
13. Fasol R, Mahdjoobian K, Joubert-Hubner E. Mitral repair in patients with severely calcified annulus: feasibility, surgery, and results. *Heart Valve Dis.* 2002;11:153–159.
14. Grossi EA, Galloway AC, Steinberg BM, et al. Severe calcification does not affect long-term outcome of mitral valve repair. *Ann Thorac Surg.* 1994;58:685–687.

Commissural Repair Techniques

10

COMMISSUROPLASTY WITH PERICARDIUM

Lai and Chard describe a commissuroplasty for a defect caused by extensive debridement of the leaflet and annulus (Fig. 10.1) (1).

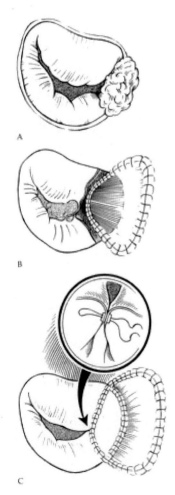

Figure 10.1 Commissuroplasty. **A:** Vegetation and abscess located in the posteromedial commissure of the mitral valve. **B:** Radical debridement of the infected annulus and adjacent leaflets resulted in a large defect in the mitral valve orifice. The annular defect was patched with pericardium. **C:** The leaflet remnants were approximated at the leading edge with a horizontal mattress suture to form a zone of apposition (**inset**). The residual D-shaped defect between the mitral annular patch and apposed leaflets was closed with a pericardial patch, thus restoring valve competence. (From Lai DT, Chard RB. Commissuroplasty: a method of valve repair for mitral and tricuspid endocarditis. *Ann Thorac Surg.* 1999;68:1727–1730.)

SLIDING LEAFLET PLASTY OR PARACOMMISURAL SLIDING PLASTY

Figures 10.2 and 10.3 show the application of the sliding plasty technique for commissural prolapse used by van Herwerden et al. (2).

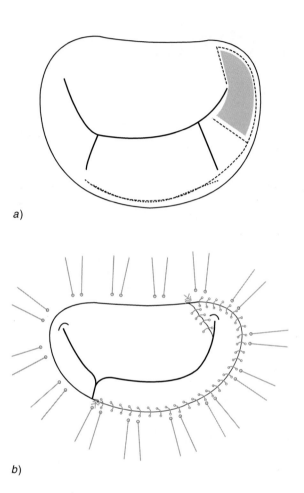

a)

b)

Figure 10.2   **A:** Incisions; dark area is resected. **B:** Completed repair. (From van Herwerden LA, Taams MA, Bos E. Repair of commissural prolapse by extended leaflet sliding. *Ann Thorac Surg.* 1994;57:387–390.)

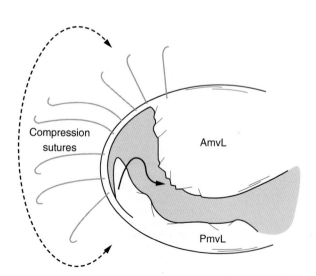

Figure 10.3   Rotation paracommissural sliding plasty. (From Ng CK, Punzengruber C, Pachinger O, et al. Valve repair in mitral regurgitation complicated by severe annulus calcification. *Ann Thorac Surg.* 2000;70:53–58.)

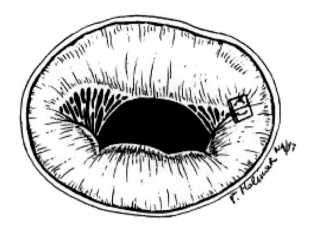

Figure 10.4 Paracommissural edge-to-edge repair. (From Maisano F, Torracca L, Oppizzi M, et al. The edge-to-edge technique: a simplified method to correct mitral insufficiency. *Eur J Cardiothorac Surg.* 1998;13:240–245.)

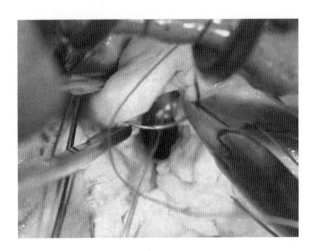

Figure 10.5 Medial commissuroplasty. (Clip 6, Case 4)

PARACOMMISSURAL EDGE-TO-EDGE REPAIR (COMMISSUROPLASTY)

A paracommissural edge-to-edge repair is a simpler procedure than sliding commissuroplasty for treating prolapse at one commissure. This can be performed with a figure-of-eight suture or a pledgeted or plain mattress suture (Fig. 10.4). This approach is quick and reliable and does not create stenosis (Fig. 10.5).

REFERENCES

1. Lai DT, Chard RB. Commissuroplasty: a method of valve repair for mitral and tricuspid endocarditis. *Ann Thorac Surg.* 1999;68:1727–1730.
2. van Herwerden LA, Taams MA, Bos E. Repair of commissural prolapse by extended leaflet sliding. *Ann Thorac Surg.* 1994;57:387–390.

Other Techniques

11

LEAFLET DEBRIDEMENT

Areas of the leaflets can be stiff and thickened commonly seen with rheumatic disease. Sharp excision of fibrous tissue and the removal of calcium can improve leaflet apposition and eliminate leaks between the leaflets.

CHORDAL LENGTHENING

For Type IIIA leaflet abnormalities papillary muscle and chordal lysis, primarily used for mitral stenosis, can be used to free the chordae, allowing increased valvular excursion (Fig. 11.1; See Fig. 7.2). This is particularly important when repairing regurgitation secondary to rheumatic disease in which chordal and papillary muscle shortening has pulled the leaflets down into the ventricle, preventing the normal doming of the leaflet and shortening the coaptation surface.

CHORDAL CUTTING RELEASE

Messas et al. described focused cutting of selected second-order chordae to the anterior leaflet to reduce regurgitation by eliminating deformation of the leaflet (or "seagull" deformity) in a sheep model of mitral regurgitation (Fig. 11.2) (1). This effect was sustained long term (2). This technique has been used clinically to release tethering of the posterior and anterior leaflets. Once bowing of the leaflet is released there is better apposition with the opposite leaflet.

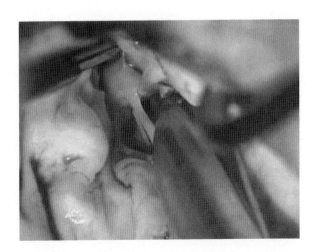

Figure 11.1   Release of secondary chordae to improve leaflet mobility. (Clip 3, Case 3)

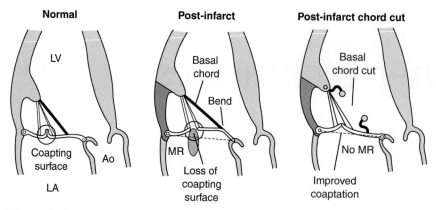

Figure 11.2   Chordal cutting to alter the shape of the leaflet. (From Messas E, Guerrero JL, Handschumacher MD, et al. Chordal cutting: a new therapeutic approach for ischemic mitral regurgitation. *Circulation*. 2001;104:1958–1963.)

POSTERIOR PAPILLARY MUSCLE RELOCATION

With chronic ischemic mitral regurgitation the posterior papillary muscle is displaced apically (3). Hung et al. documented, in an animal model, that simple repositioning of the bulging posterior wall and associated papillary muscle into the ventricle with associated reduction of apical traction of the mitral leaflets reversed mitral regurgitation (4). This reversal was demonstrated in a sheep model with posterior suture plication (Fig. 11.3) (5).

This principle was applied by Kron et al., who detailed a technique to promote repair in the presence of a Carpentier Type IIIb leaflet abnormality caused by tethering of the leaflets to the posterior papillary muscle with resultant traction into the ventricle (6). As the annulus may not be dilated, annuloplasty alone may not correct the regurgitation. They performed this repair by passing a 3-0 polypropylene suture twice through the fibrous portion of the posterior papillary muscle then through the annulus just posterior to the right fibrous trigone (Fig. 11.4). Once the annuloplasty ring was in place, tension on this relocat-

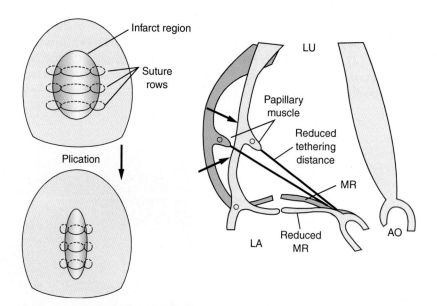

Figure 11.3   Posterior suture plication to reposition the papillary muscle. (From Liel-Cohen N, Guerrero JL, Otsuji Y, et al. Design of a new surgical approach for ventricular remodeling to relieve ischemic mitral regurgitation: insights from 3-dimensional echocardiography. *Circulation*. 2000;101:2756–2763.)

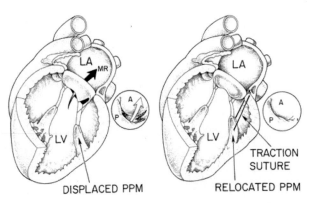

Figure 11.4 Posterior papillary muscle relocation for Type IIIb abnormality. (From Kron IL, Green R, Cope JT. Surgical relocation of the posterior papillary muscle in chronic ischemic mitral regurgitation. *Ann Thorac Surg.* 2002;74:600–601.)

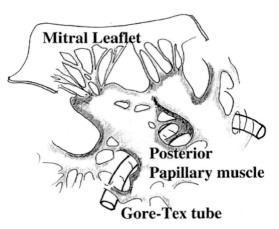

Figure 11.5 Gore-Tex® tube encircling the trabecular base of the posterior and anterior papillary muscle, tightened and secured with sutures to bring the papillary muscles into close contact. (From Hvass U, Tapia M, Baron F, Pouzet B, Shafy A. Papillary muscle sling: a new functional approach to mitral repair in patients with ischemic left ventricular dysfunction and functional mitral regurgitation. *Ann Thorac Surg.* 2003;75:809–811.)

ing suture was adjusted to maximize leaflet coaptation. They reported excellent early results in 18 patients. However, given the significant stress placed on the papillary muscle, Carpentier expressed concern about the long-term durability of this approach (A. Carpentier, personal communication).

PAPILLARY MUSCLE SLING

An alternative technique for reducing posterior papillary muscle displacement was described by Hvass et al. (7). They created a papillary muscle sling using a 4-mm Gore-Tex® tube graft to pull the papillary muscles together to complement the support of an annuloplasty ring (Fig. 11.5). They demonstrated a reduction in the tenting effect from 14 ± 2.8 millimeters to 4 ± 1.41 millimeters.

CHORDAL SHORTENING

Chordal shortening procedures at the level of the papillary muscle are discussed here for historical significance, and to recommend against future application. This technique was described by Carpentier (8) and involved burying the elongated chord in a slit made in the papillary muscle as depicted in Figure 11.6. Smedira et al. reviewed their results and noted a 5-year actuarial freedom from reoperation of 96% after chordal transfer (discussed below) (posterior leaflet transfer [75%], transfer of a secondary chorda [21%], or both [3%] to the free edge of the anterior leaflet) and 74% after chordal shortening, $p = 0.003$, noting that chordal shortening was an independent predictor of reoperation (9). This was confirmed by El Khoury et al. (10) and Fucci et al. (11). The failure mode noted for this repair is depicted in Figure 11.7.

In response to this, Fundaro et al. updated the results of their chordal shortening technique with a technique described as "free edge remodeling" (12), (see Chapter 8, Figs. 8.4, 8.5). Here they present a slight alteration in the technique for chordal shortening demonstrated in Fig. 11.8. They reported a 3.2% reoperation rate for recurrent prolapse at 16.8 months.

An alternative chordal shortening technique was described by Duran wherein the papillary muscle head is repositioned (13) (Figs. 11.9 and 11.10). Similar to this is the papillary

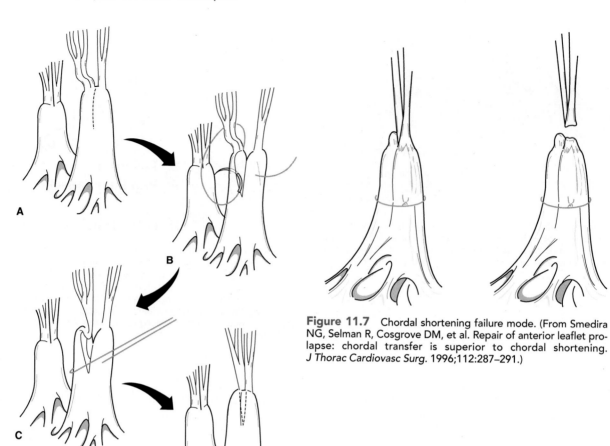

Figure 11.6 Technique of chordal shortening. (From Muehrcke DD, Cosgrove DM. Mitral valvuloplasty. In: Edmunds, Jr. LH, ed. *Cardiac Surgery in the Adult.* New York: McGraw-Hill, 1997:1006.)

Figure 11.7 Chordal shortening failure mode. (From Smedira NG, Selman R, Cosgrove DM, et al. Repair of anterior leaflet prolapse: chordal transfer is superior to chordal shortening. *J Thorac Cardiovasc Surg.* 1996;112:287–291.)

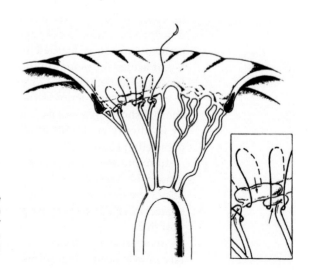

Figure 11.8 Technique of chordal suture plication and free edge remodeling, compare to Figures 8.4 and 8.5. (From Fundaro P, Lemma M, Di Mattia DG, Santoli C. Repair of anterior leaflet prolapse: chordal transfer versus chordal shortening. Which is better? *J Thorac Cardiovasc Surg.* 1997;114: 1125–1127.)

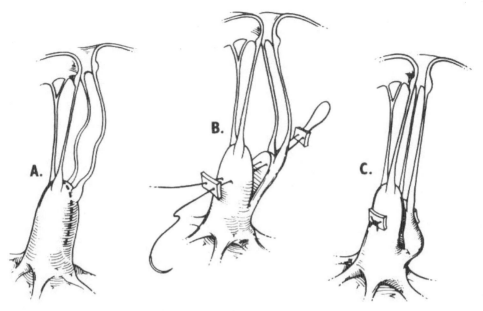

Figure 11.9 Chordal shortening by papillary muscle sliding plasty. (From Duran CMG. Surgical techniques for the repair of anterior mitral leaflet prolapse. *J Card Surg*. 1999:14;471–481.)

muscle repositioning described by Dreyfus et al. as an alternative to chordal shortening with similar long-term results (Fig. 11.11) (14).

PAPILLARY MUSCLE SHORTENING

Fasol et al. described a technique of papillary muscle shortening when the head became fibrotic and elongated causing prolapse and regurgitation (Fig. 11.12) (15). This technique was used to repair the valve in 88 patients with no failures on short-term follow-up.

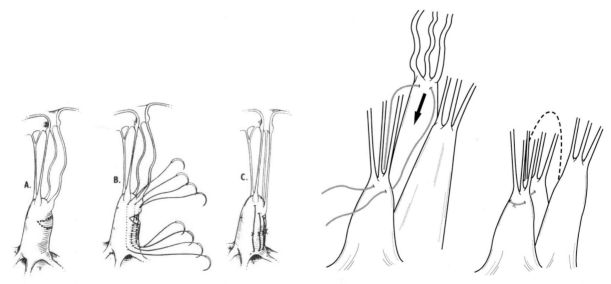

Figure 11.10 Chordal shortening by papillary muscle head repositioning. (From Duran CMG. Surgical techniques for the repair of anterior mitral leaflet prolapse. *J Card Surg*. 1999:14;471–481.)

Figure 11.11 Posterior papillary muscle repositioning. (From Dreyfus GD, Bahrami T, Alayle N, et al. Repair of anterior leaflet prolapse by papillary muscle repositioning: a new surgical option. *Ann Thorac Surg*. 2001:71:1464–1470.)

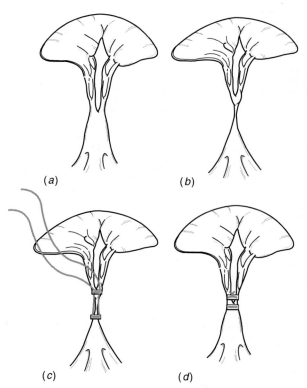

(a)   (b)

(c)   (d)

Figure 11.12 Papillary muscle shortening. **A:** Normal, **B:** Elongated and fibrotic, **C:** repair suture placed, **D:** repair suture tied. (From Fasol R, Wild T, Pfannmuller B, Stumpf J, Hacker R. Papillary muscle shortening for mitral valve reconstruction in patients with ischemic mitral insufficiency. *Eur Heart J.* 1998;19:1730–1744.)

CHORDAL TRANSPOSITION OR TRANSFER

Two types of chordal transposition have been described: Transposition of a primary posterior leaflet chorda to the edge of the anterior leaflet and transposition of an anterior leaflet secondary chorda to the leaflet edge.

Transposition of a primary posterior leaflet chordae (also referred to as the flip-over technique (16) was described by Carpentier (8). This involves quadrangular resection of a portion of the posterior leaflet and primary closure, with transposition to the underside of the flail segment of the anterior leaflet (Fig. 11.13). Utilizing this technique in 39 patients,

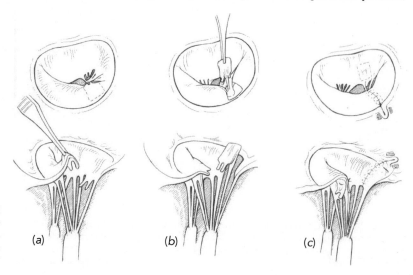

Figure 11.13 Posterior chordal transfer. (From Muehrcke DD, Cosgrove DM. Mitral valvuloplasty. In: Edmunds, Jr. LH, ed. *Cardiac Surgery in the Adult.* New York: McGraw-Hill. 1997:1007.)

(a)   (b)   (c)

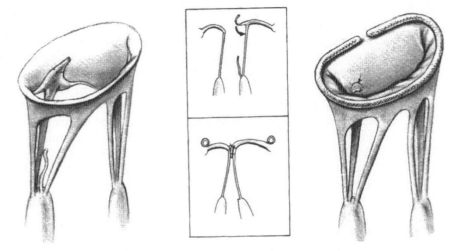

Figure 11.14 Fixation of leaflet edge to secondary chorda. (From Carpentier A. Cardiac valve surgery—the "French Correction." *J Thorac Cardiovasc Surg.* 1983;86: 323–337.)

Lessana et al. reported a 97.4 ± 5.2% freedom from reoperation rate at 4 years (17). Similar results were reported by Salati et al.: 91.5 ± 5.2% in 48 patients at 3 years (18,19), Sousa Uva et al. (20), and Smedira et al. (9).

Use of a secondary chorda to secure the leaflet edge was described by Carpentier who fixed the leaflet edge to the secondary chorda as demonstrated in Figure 11.14 (8). The transposition variant of this is shown in Figure 11.15.

A note of caution is raised by Nielsen et al. who reported that in a sheep model, isolated division of an anterior leaflet secondary chordae resulted in regional left ventricular systolic dysfunction near the insertion site (21). The clinical implications of this observation for mitral repair are unclear.

CHORDAL REPLACEMENT

Chordal replacement to correct anterior leaflet prolapse has been described as an alternative to shortening or transposition. Gregory et al. described a technique used in two patients in which

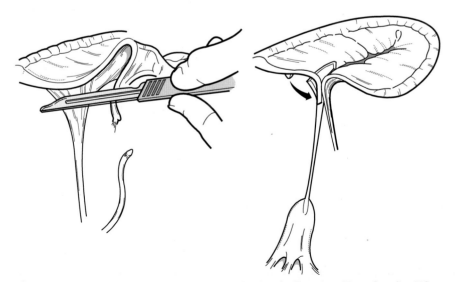

Figure 11.15 Transposition of secondary chord to leaflet edge. (From Smedira NG, Selman R, Cosgrove DM, et al. Repair of anterior leaflet prolapse: chordal transfer is superior to chordal shortening. *J Thorac Cardiovasc Surg.* 1996;112:287–291.)

a strip of leaflet from the anterior leaflet was sewn to the papillary muscle (Fig. 11.16) (22). Though an interesting technique, no long-term follow-up or reports of its utilization in additional patients could be found. Given the availability of other techniques with documented success application of this technique cannot be recommended.

The use of various prosthetic materials has been reported to replace the damaged or diseased chordae, including expanded polytetrafluoroethylene (PTFE) (23,24) and glutaraldehyde-tanned xenograft pericardium (24), both demonstrating excellent long-term durability. The PTFE becomes covered with a normal fibrosa and intima and retains flexibility (25). Eishi et al. found pericardium to be inferior to PTFE and recommended against its use (26).

A number of techniques for the insertion of PTFE chordae have been published (13) (Figs. 11.17–11.20). The suture should be tied so the body of the leaflet is at the level of the annular plane (27) (Figs. 11.21–11.24).

David reviewed his experience in 1998: Of 324 repairs performed, he utilized PTFE chordae in 165 (Figs. 11.25–11.27). He noted no negative effect on long-term outcome with their use and felt that he was able to expand the number of valves repaired utilizing these techniques (28). Zussa et al. have confirmed these results (29,30). Chordal replacement has demonstrated superior long-term results in comparison to chordal shortening (31).

Technical Details

Most authors recommend 4-0 or 5-0 PTFE suture, though one recently espoused the use of 2-0, claiming that 5-0 was too weak. Determining the proper length for artificial chordae can be challenging. As Frater points out, successful achievement of ideal length for the new chordae is influenced by accurate determination of the length (the ideal length may differ from that determined in the flaccid heart) and accurately tying the knot (PTFE is slippery) (32).

A number of techniques have been described to determine appropriate length, including using tourniquets to adjust the length after the other aspects of the repair are complete (Fig. 11.28) (33). Adams et al. advocate using a surgeon's knot with saline testing to adjust the leaflet height instead of tourniquets and pledgets (Fig. 11.29), again, after the rest of the repair is completed (34). Sarsam advocates a different technique that can be applied with multiple areas of unileaflet and bileaflet prolapse. A temporary figure-of-eight suture is used to reapproximate the leaflet edges then the chordal suture, which was brought up

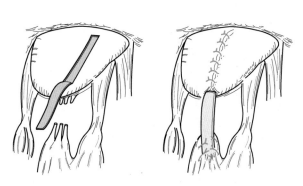

Figure 11.16 Anterior leaflet strip to treat prolapse. (From Gregory F Jr, Takeda R, Silva S, Facanha L, Meier MA. A new technique for repair of mitral insufficiency caused by ruptured chordae of the anterior leaflet. *J Thorac Cardiovasc Surg.* 1988;96:765–768.)

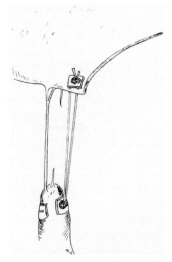

Figure 11.17 Technique for insertion of Gore-Tex® chord using glutaraldehyde fixed pericardial pledgets. This approach has the disadvantage that the tied suture may impinge on the area of leaflet apposition. (From Zussa C. Different applications of ePTFE valve chordae: surgical technique. *J Heart Valve Dis.* 1996 Jul;5(4):356–361.)

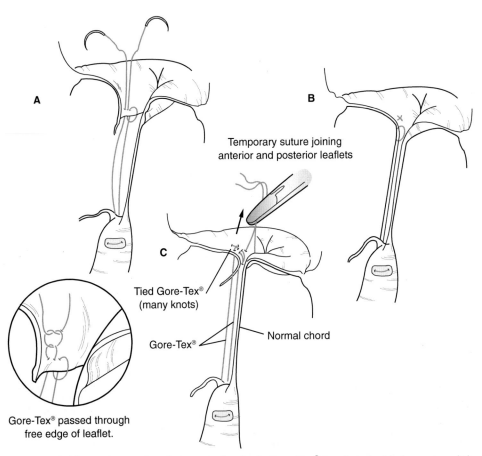

Figure 11.18 Technique for placement of a single Gore-Tex®chord. A double loop around the leaflet edge rolls it under and prevents slippage while tying. (From Duran CMG. Surgical techniques for the repair of anterior mitral leaflet prolapse. *J Card Surg* 1999;14:471–481.)

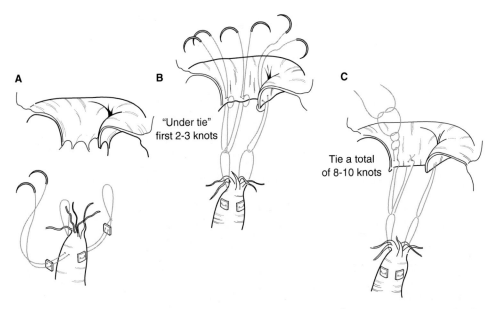

Figure 11.19 Technique for placement of a multiple Gore-Tex®chords. (From Duran CMG. Surgical techniques for the repair of anterior mitral leaflet prolapse. *J Card Surg.* 1999;14:471–481.)

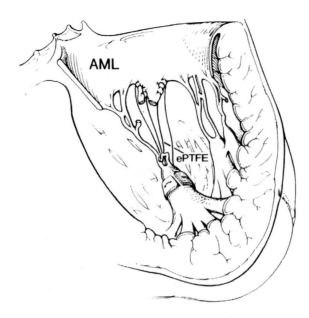

Figure 11.20 Alternative method of suturing to the leaflet edge below the plane of the valve coaptation. (From Phillips MR, Daly RC, Schaff HV, et al. Repair of anterior leaflet mitral valve prolapse: chordal replacement versus chordal shortening. *Ann Thorac Surg.* 2000;69:25–29.)

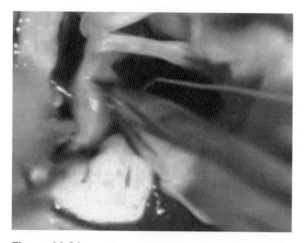

Figure 11.21 Anchoring the PTFE suture in the papillary muscle. (Clip 3, Case 4)

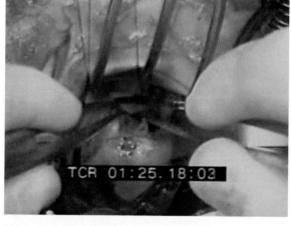

Figure 11.22 Anchoring the PTFE suture in the anterior papillary muscle. (Clip 3, Case 6)

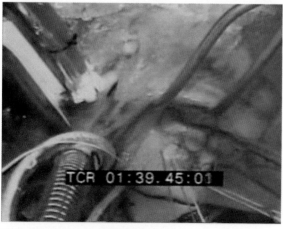

Figure 11.23 Attachment of the PTFE suture to the anterior leaflet. (Clip 6, Case 6)

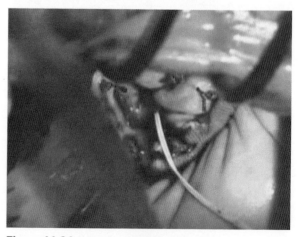

Figure 11.24 Attachment of the PTFE suture to the anterior leaflet. (Clip 8, Case 4)

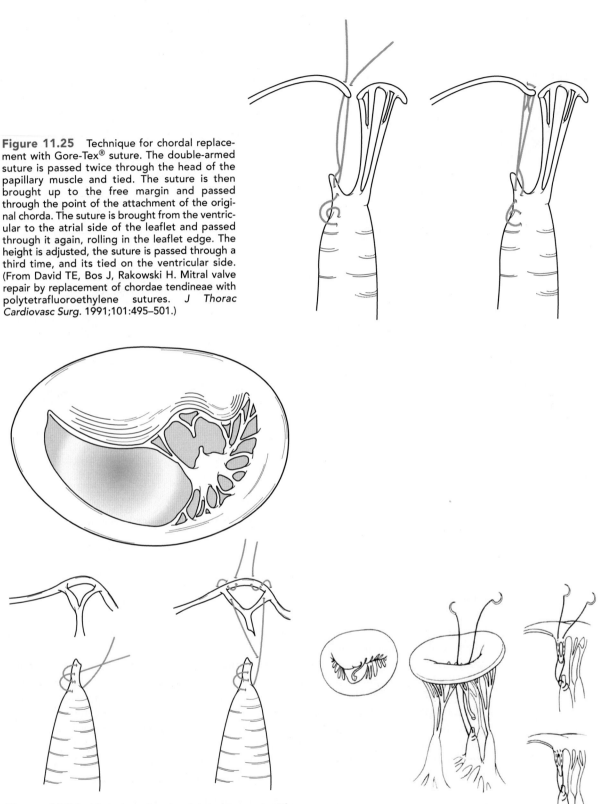

Figure 11.25 Technique for chordal replacement with Gore-Tex® suture. The double-armed suture is passed twice through the head of the papillary muscle and tied. The suture is then brought up to the free margin and passed through the point of the attachment of the original chorda. The suture is brought from the ventricular to the atrial side of the leaflet and passed through it again, rolling in the leaflet edge. The height is adjusted, the suture is passed through a third time, and its tied on the ventricular side. (From David TE, Bos J, Rakowski H. Mitral valve repair by replacement of chordae tendineae with polytetrafluoroethylene sutures. *J Thorac Cardiovasc Surg.* 1991;101:495–501.)

Figure 11.26 Technique for chordal replacement with Gore-Tex® suture. Similar to the technique in Figure 11.25 but for a wider segment of prolapse or to replace two adjacent chordae. Each segment of the suture is passed through the anchor point and run toward the other, avoiding crimping of the leaflet. (From David TE, Bos J, Rakowski H. Mitral valve repair by replacement of chordae tendineae with polytetrafluoroethylene sutures. *J Thorac Cardiovasc Surg.* 1991;101: 495–501.)

Figure 11.27 Alternative technique for chordae replacement with PTFE. (From David TE, Omran A, Armstrong S, Sun Z, Ivanov J. Long-term results of mitral valve repair for myxomatous disease with and without chordal replacement with expanded polytetrafluoroethylene sutures. *J Thorac Cardiovasc Surg.* 1998;115:1279–1285.)

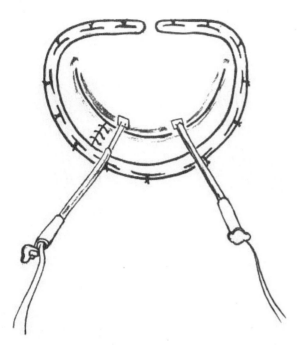

Figure 11.28 Technique for determining ideal length of artificial chordae. (From Kasegawa H, Kamata S, Hirata S, et al. Simple method for determining proper length of artificial chordae in mitral valve repair. *Ann Thorac Surg.* 1994;57: 237–238.)

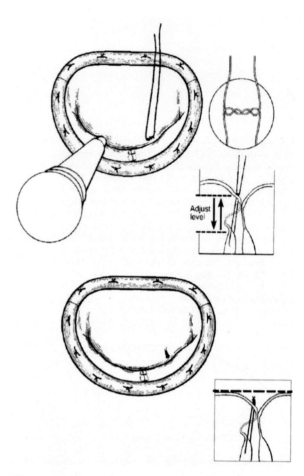

Figure 11.29 Technique for optimizing length of the artificial chordae using a surgeon's knot to avoid slippage. (From Adams DH, Kadner A, Chen RH. Artificial mitral valve chordae replacement made simple. *Ann Thorac Surg.* 2001; 71:1377–1388.)

through the rough portion of the valve, is tied with three knots to secure it, then looped again through the leaflet to secure it in place (Fig. 11.30) (35). In the case of bileaflet prolapse, the first suture is tied to approximate the plane of the mitral annulus then used as a reference for tying the remaining artificial chordal sutures. In contrast, Rankin recommends using a removable hemoclip to secure the suture during testing, then tying on the clips when the correct height is determined (36). Reimink et al., using a finite element model demonstrated that the ideal length of artificial chordae should be the same as or longer than the replaced chordae to optimize function and stress in the repaired valve (37).

Techniques to prevent slippage while tying the suture include grasping the suture with a clamp or hemoclip at the cusp edge level (33) or passing the suture through the free edge several times to create friction and prevent slippage (32) (Figs. 11.31 and 11.32). If a clip is used, the suture can be tied against a clip and then the clip can be removed.

PTFE Chordal Replacement for Isolated Posterior Leaflet Prolapse

The use of PTFE to repair posterior leaflet prolapse as an alternative to excision of the P2 scallop has been described (38). Rather than excising the flail leaflet it is reattached to the papillary muscle. This may be easier than and just as effective as more complicated approaches (Fig. 11.33). Sutures may be necessary to secure the posterior leaflet and prevent prolapse after a sliding or folding plasty (Fig. 11.34).

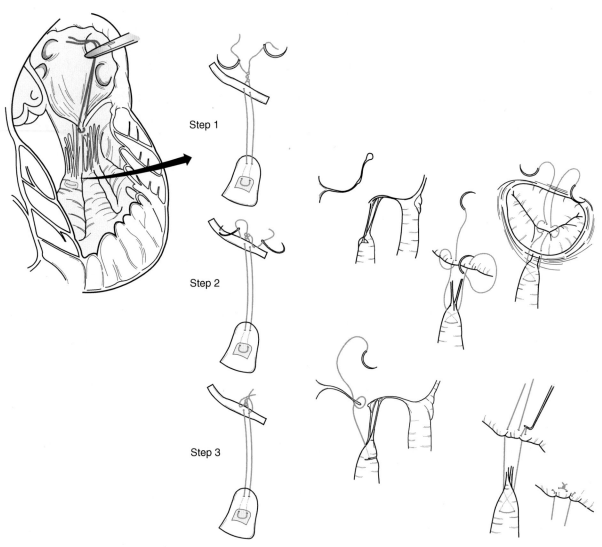

Figure 11.30 Technique to optimize length of artificial choral sutures. (From Sarsam MA. Simplified technique for determining the length of artificial chordae in mitral valve repair. *Ann Thorac Surg.* 2002;73:1659–1660.)

Step 1

Step 2

Step 3

Figure 11.31 Chordal replacement with 4-0 PTFE suture. (From Chitwood Jr. WR. Mitral valve repair: ischemic. In: Kaiser LR, Kron IL, Spray TL. *Mastery of Cardiothoracic Surgery.* Philadelphia: Lippincott-Raven. 1998:320.)

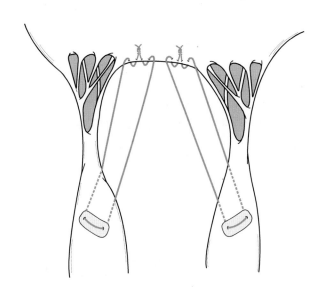

Figure 11.32 Use of 5-0 PTFE to create artificial chordae. (From Kobayashi J, Sasako Y, Bando K. Ten-year experience of chordal replacement with expanded polytetrafluoroethylene in mitral valve repair. *Circulation.* 2000;102:III–30.)

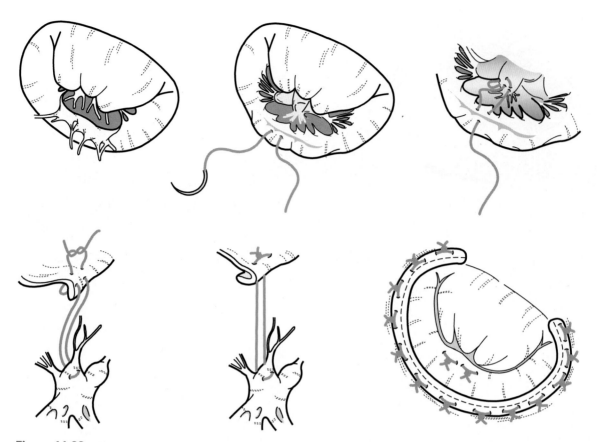

Figure 11.33   Repair of posterior leaflet prolapse with a PTFE replacement chord. (From Nigro JJ, Schwartz DS, Bart RD, et al. Neochordal repair of the posterior mitral leaflet. *J Thorac Cardiovasc Surg.* 2004;127:440–447.)

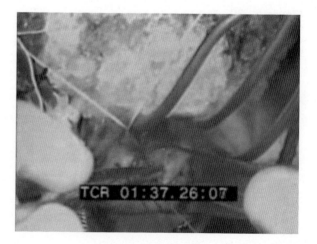

Figure 11.34   Securing the posterior leaflet. (Clip 5, Case 6)

POSTERIOR TRICUSPID LEAFLET AUTOTRANSPLANT

Gregori et al. described the use of a portion of the tricuspid valve, a portion of the anterior leaflet in one case, and the whole posterior leaflet in the second case (39). They present longer-term results in 20 patients (40). They report 90% freedom from reoperation, the reoperations were not related to failure of the grafted tricuspid valve. Sixteen of 17 patients evaluated by echocardiography had no or mild mitral regurgitation (Fig. 11.35). These results were confirmed by others (41,42). Given the successful use of artificial chords, this procedure seems unnecessarily complex.

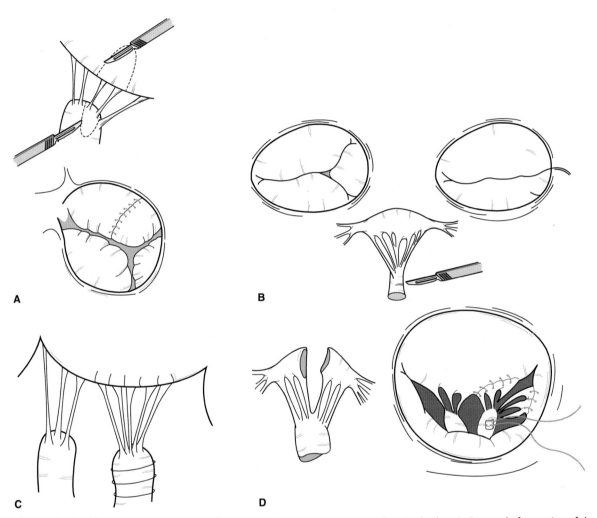

Figure 11.35 Technique of grafting a portion of the tricuspid valve to repair the mitral valve. **A:** Removal of a portion of the anterior leaflet of the tricuspid valve. **B:** Removal of the posterior leaflet of the tricuspid valve. **C:** Repair of the anterior leaflet of the mitral valve. **D:** Repair of the mitral commissure. (**A and C:** from Gregori Jr. F, da Silva SS, Goulart MP, et al. Grafting of chordae tendineae: a new technique for the repair of mitral insufficiency caused by ruptured chordae of the anterior leaflet. *J Thorac Cardiovasc Surg.* 1994; 107:635-638. **B and D:** from Gregori F Jr, Cordeiro CO, Croti UA, et al. Partial tricuspid valve transfer for repair of mitral insufficiency due to ruptured chordae tendineae. *Ann Thorac Surg.* 1999;68:1686–1691.)

PAPILLARY MUSCLE REPAIR

Papillary muscle rupture can be partial or complete. Partial rupture can present as chronic mitral regurgitation, complete rupture is generally so symptomatic that immediate surgery is required. Acute complete rupture is often associated with extensive infarction and difficult to repair. Repair can be attempted using pledgeted sutures passed through the papillary muscle

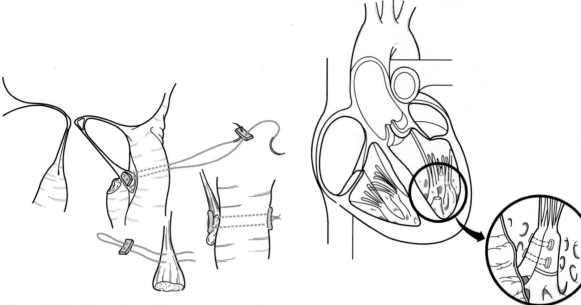

Figure 11.36   Repair of complete rupture by suture to the ventricle. (From Chitwood Jr. WR. Mitral valve repair: ischemic. In: Kaiser LR, Kron IL, Spray TL. *Mastery of Cardiothoracic Surgery.* Philadelphia: Lippincott-Raven. 1998:318.)

Figure 11.37   Repair of rupture of one head of the papillary muscle. (From Muehrcke DD, Cosgrove DM. Mitral valvuloplasty. In: Edmunds, Jr. LH, ed. *Cardiac Surgery in the Adult.* New York: McGraw-Hill, 1997:1011.)

then through the ventricular wall (Fig. 11.36). Partial rupture or rupture of one head can be repaired in the acute or chronic situation by attaching the ruptured head to the adjacent head with pledgeted suture (Fig. 11.37). Fasol et al. demonstrated good results in 6 patients (43).

EDGE-TO-EDGE OR DOUBLE ORIFICE REPAIR

The group headed by Alfieri described, refined, and provided follow-up on the use of the edge-to-edge repair to treat prolapse of one of the mitral leaflets (Fig. 11.38) (44–47). The overall five-year freedom from reoperation when used with an annuloplasty procedure was 92 ± 3.4% (46). In contrast, Lorusso et al. noted an 80% freedom from reoperation at 8 years (when used alone and with other repair techniques). Risk factors for failure included left ventricular dysfunction, pulmonary arterial hypertension, marked left atrial enlargement, and pericardial annuloplasty (48). Patients with the edge-to-edge repair had smaller valve orifices with no significant stenosis identified (45,49). This has also been applied for poor coaptation in Type IIIB leaflet abnormality (50). Some advocate this over other techniques for its ease of use (51,52). No significant stenosis was created with a combination of the edge-to-edge repair with ring annuloplasty (53).

This repair technique has also been applied via the transaortic approach (Fig. 11.39) (54). This technique has also been applied to eliminate residual regurgitation after the use of traditional repair techniques (55).

LEAFLET REPLACEMENT OR AUGMENTATION WITH PERICARDIUM

Glutaraldehyde-preserved and untreated autologous pericardium has been used to replace or augment leaflets as part of the valve repair (56). For preservation, the pericardium is harvested and treated in 0.62% glutaraldehyde-buffered solution at room temperature for 15 minutes and rinsed in saline for an additional 15 minutes. Techniques include straddling endoventricular pericardial patch annuloplasty (as discussed above for the severely calcified annulus); patch as a substitute for the posterior leaflet (used to bridge the gap between the leaflet remnants and the annulus); paracommissural extension patch plasty (to fill the commissural area and approximate the two leaflet remnants); posterior leaflet extension patch plasty (to increase the posterior leaflet surface area by more than 50% by inserting a patch between the leaflet and the annulus); patch as substitute for or to enlarge the anterior leaflet (a circular pericardial patch to repair a defect); and chordal replacement (57) (Fig. 11.40). The technique of anterior leaflet extension has recently been recommended as a compliment to myectomy for hypertrophic obstructive cardiomyopathy, the enlarged anterior leaflet moving the point of coaptation away from the septum (58). The gluteraldehyde-treated pericardium has proven to be durable, remains pliable, and does not become excessively calcified (57). Reports using untreated autologous pericardium have produced variable results, often related to shrinkage or calcification of the pericardium (59). Sauvage first reported the use of autologous pericardium in 1966 to augment the surface area or "advance the leaflet" (60,61). Chauvaud et al. reported 64 patients who underwent leaflet extension of the mitral valve between 1980 and 1989 (62). This technique was applied most commonly with regurgitation secondary to rheumatic fever (69%), other causes including bacterial endocarditis (17%), congenital (8%), endomyocardial fibrosis (4.5%), and trauma (1.5%). Follow-up extended from 6 months to 9 years (mean 3.1 ± 2.5 years). Six patients (12%) who underwent reoperation for progression of rheumatic disease; no failures related to the pericardium were noted and there was no evidence of calcification of the pericardial patch. Mitral valve insufficiency was trivial or absent in 80% of the patients.

Kincaid reported a small but encouraging series using anterior leaflet augmentation to compensate for excess posterior leaflet retraction in ischemic mitral regurgitation (Fig. 11.41) (63).

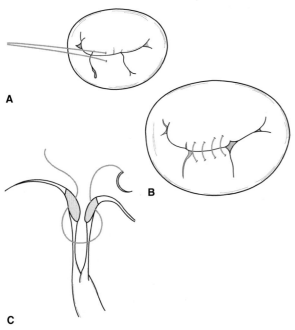

Figure 11.38 "Edge-to-edge" repair technique for anterior leaflet prolapse. **A:** Central stitch to check symmetry. **B:** Completed running suture creating the repair. **C:** Side view demonstrating suture placement through the rough zone of the mitral leaflets. (From Maisano F, Schreuder JJ, Oppizzi M, et al. The double-orifice technique as a standardized approach to treat mitral regurgitation due to severe myxomatous disease: surgical technique. *Eur J Cardiothorac Surg.* 2000;17:201–205.)

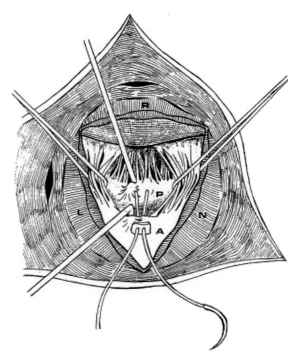

Figure 11.39 Transaortic approach for edge-to-edge repair. Care must be taken to ensure the suture is placed centrally in both leaflets. (From Kallner G, van der Linden J, Hadjinikolaou L, Lindblom D. Transaortic approach for the Alfieri stitch. *Ann Thorac Surg.* 2001;71:378–379.)

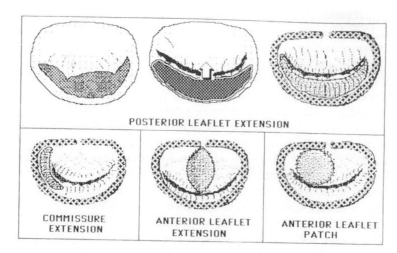

POSTERIOR LEAFLET EXTENSION

COMMISSURE
EXTENSION

ANTERIOR LEAFLET
EXTENSION

ANTERIOR LEAFLET
PATCH

Figure 11.40 Various techniques for patching the mitral valve with gluter-aldehyde-preserved pericardium. (From Chauvaud S, Jebara V, Chachques JC, et al. Valve extension with glutaraldehyde-preserved autologous pericardium. Results in mitral valve repair. *J Thorac Cardiovasc Surg.* 1991;102:171–177.)

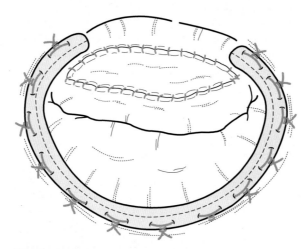

Figure 11.41 Anterior leaflet augmentation for ischemic mitral regurgitation. (From Kincaid EH, Riley RD, Hines MH, Hammon JW, Kon ND. Anterior leaflet augmentation for ischemic mitral regurgitation. *Ann Thorac Surg.* 2004;78: 564–568).

REFERENCES

1. Messas E, Guerrero JL, Handschumacher MD, et al. Chordal cutting: a new therapeutic approach for ischemic mitral regurgitation. *Circulation.* 2001;104:1958–1963.
2. Messas E, Pouzet B, Touchot B, et al. Efficacy of chordal cutting to relieve chronic persistent ischemic mitral regurgitation. *Circulation.* 2003;108 Suppl 1:II;111–115.
3. Kumanohoso T, Otsuji Y, Yoshifuku S, et al. Mechanism of higher incidence of ischemic mitral regurgitation in patients with inferior myocardial infarction: quantitative analysis of left ventricular and mitral valve geometry in 103 patients with prior myocardial infarction. *J Thorac Cardiovasc Surg.* 2003;125:135–143.
4. Hung J, Guerrero JL, Handschumacher MD, Supple G, et al. Reverse ventricular remodeling reduces ischemic mitral regurgitation. Echo-guided device application in the beating heart. *Circulation.* 2002;106:2594.
5. Liel-Cohen N, Guerrero JL, Otsuji Y, et al. Design of a new surgical approach for ventricular remodeling to relieve ischemic mitral regurgitation: insights from 3-dimensional echocardiography. *Circulation.* 2000;101:2756–2763.
6. Kron IL, Green R, Cope JT. Surgical relocation of the posterior papillary muscle in chronic ischemic mitral regurgitation. *Ann Thorac Surg.* 2002;74:600–601.
7. Hvass U, Tapia M, Baron F, Pouzet B, Shafy A. Papillary muscle sling: a new functional approach to mitral repair in patients with ischemic left ventricular dysfunction and functional mitral regurgitation. *Ann Thorac Surg.* 2003; 75:809–811.
8. Carpentier A. Cardiac Valve Surgery—the "French Correction." *J Thorac Cardiovasc Surg.* 1983;86:323–337.
9. Smedira NG, Selman R, Cosgrove DM, et al. Repair of anterior leaflet prolapse: chordal transfer is superior to chordal shortening. *J Thorac Cardiovasc Surg.* 1996;112:287–291.

10. El Khoury G, Noirhomme F, Verhelst R, Rubay J, Dion R. Surgical repair of the prolapsing anterior leaflet in degenerative mitral valve disease. *J Heart Valve Dis.* 2000;9:75–80.
11. Fucci C, Sandrelli L, Pardini A, et al. Improved results with mitral valve repair using new surgical techniques. *Eur J Cardiothorac Surg.* 1995;9:621–626.
12. Fundaro P, Lemma M, Di Mattia DG, Santoli C. Repair of anterior leaflet prolapse: chordal transfer versus chordal shortening. Which is better? *J Thorac Cardiovasc Surg.* 1997;114:1125–1127.
13. Duran CMG. Surgical techniques for the repair of anterior mitral leaflet prolapse. *J Card Surg.* 1999;14:471–481.
14. Dreyfus GD, Bahrami T, Alayle N, et al. Repair of anterior leaflet prolapse by papillary muscle repositioning: a new surgical option. *Ann Thorac Surg.* 2001;71:1464–1470.
15. Fasol R, Lakew F, Pfannmuller B, Slepian MJ, Joubert-Hubner E. Papillary muscle repair surgery in ischemic mitral valve patients. *Ann Thorac Surg.* 2000;70:771–776.
16. Duran CG. Repair of anterior mitral leaflet chordal rupture or elongation (the flip-over technique). *J Card Surg.* 1986;1:161–166.
17. Lessana A, Carbone C, Romano M, et al. Mitral valve repair: results and the decision-making process in reconstruction. Report of 275 cases. *J Thorac Cardiovasc Surg.* 1990;99:622–630.
18. Salati M, Scrofani R, Fundaro P, Cialfi A, Santoli C. Correction of anterior mitral prolapse. Results of chordal transposition. *J Thorac Cardiovasc Surg.* 1992;104:1268–1273.
19. Salati M, Moriggia S, Scrofani R, Santoli C. Chordal transposition for anterior mitral prolapse: early and long-term results. *Eur J Cardiothorac Surg.* 1997;11:268–273.
20. Sousa Uva M, Grare P, Jebara V, et al. Transposition of chordae in mitral valve repair. Mid-term results. *Circulation.* 1993;88:II35–38.
21. Nielsen SL, Timek TA, Green GR, et al. Influence of anterior mitral leaflet second-order chordae tendineae on left ventricular systolic function. *Circulation.* 2003;108:486–491.
22. Gregory F Jr, Takeda R, Silva S, Facanha L, Meier MA. A new technique for repair of mitral insufficiency caused by ruptured chordae of the anterior leaflet. *J Thorac Cardiovasc Surg.* 1988;96:765–768.
23. David TE. Replacement of chordae tendineae with expanded polytetrafluoroethylene sutures. *J Card Surg.* 1990;5:152–153.
24. Frater RW, Vetter HO, Zussa C, Dahm M. Chordal replacement in mitral valve repair. *Circulation.* 1990;82:IV 125–130.
25. Kobayashi J, Sasako Y, Bando K, et al. Ten-year experience of chordal replacement with expanded polytetrafluoroethylene in mitral valve repair. *Circulation.* 2000;102:III 30–34.
26. Eishi K, Kawazoe K, Nakano K, et al. Long-term results of artificial chordae implantation in patients with mitral valve prolapse. *J Heart Valve Dis.* 1997;6:594–598.
27. Duran CMG, Pekar Filip. Techniques for ensuring the correct length of new mitral chords. *J Heart Valve Dis.* 2003;12:156–161.
28. David TE, Omran A, Armstrong S, Sun Z, Ivanov J. Long-term results of mitral valve repair for myxomatous disease with and without chordal replacement with expanded polytetrafluoroethylene sutures. *J Thorac Cardiovasc Surg.* 1998;115:1279–1285.
29. Zussa C, Polesel E, Da Col U, Galloni M, Valfre C. Seven-year experience with chordal replacement with expanded polytetrafluoroethylene in floppy mitral valve. *J Thorac Cardiovasc Surg.* 1994;108:37–41.
30. Zussa C, Polesel E, Rocco F, Valfre C. Artificial chordae in the treatment of anterior mitral leaflet pathology. *Cardiovasc Surg.* 1997;5:125–128.
31. Phillips MR, Daly RC, Schaff HV, et al. Repair of anterior leaflet mitral valve prolapse: chordal replacement versus chordal shortening. *Ann Thorac Surg.* 2000;69:25–29.
32. Frater RWM. Invited commentary. *Ann Thorac Surg.* 1994;57:238–239.
33. Kasegawa H, Kamata S, Hirata S, et al. Simple method for determining proper length of artificial chordae in mitral valve repair. *Ann Thorac Surg.* 1994;57:237–238.
34. Adams DH, Kadner A, Chen RH. Artificial mitral valve chordae replacement made simple. *Ann Thorac Surg.* 2001;71:1377–378.
35. Sarsam MA. Simplified technique for determining the length of artificial chordae in mitral valve repair. *Ann Thorac Surg.* 2002;73:1659–1660.
36. Rankin JS, Orozco RE. Mitral valve repair for Barlow's Syndrome using adjustable artificial chordal replacement. Surgical Motion Pictures. Society of Thoracic Surgeons 40th Meeting. San Antonio 2004.
37. Reimink MS, Kunzelman KS, Cochran RP. The effect of chordal replacement suture length on function and stresses in repaired mitral valves: a finite element study. *J Heart Valve Dis.* 1996;5(4):365–375.
38. Nigro JJ, Schwartz DS, Bart RD, et al. Neochordal repair of the posterior mitral leaflet. *J Thorac Cardiovasc Surg.* 2004;127:440–447.
39. Gregori F Jr, da Silva SS, Goulart MP, Canesin O, Hayashi SS. Grafting of chordae tendineae: a new technique for the repair of mitral insufficiency caused by ruptured chordae of the anterior leaflet. *J Thorac Cardiovasc Surg.* 1994;107:635–638.
40. Gregori F Jr, Cordeiro CO, Croti UA, et al. Partial tricuspid valve transfer for repair of mitral insufficiency due to ruptured chordae tendineae. *Ann Thorac Surg.* 1999;68:1686–1691.
41. Khoury GE, d'Udekem Y, Noirhomme P, et al. Transfer of the posterior leaflet of the tricuspid valve to the mitral valve. *J Heart Valve Dis.* 2000;9:350–352.
42. Hvass U. Tricuspid autograft for repair of a destroyed mitral commissure. *Semin Thorac Cardiovasc Surg.* 2001;13(4 Suppl 1):43–47.
43. Fasol R, Lakew F, Wetter S. Mitral repair in patients with a ruptured papillary muscle. *Am Heart J.* 2000;139:549–554.
44. Fucci C, Sandrelli L, Pardini A, Torracca L, Ferrari M, Alfieri O. Improved results with mitral valve repair using new surgical techniques. *Eur J Cardiothorac Surg.* 1995;9:621–626.
45. Maisano F, Torracca L, Oppizzi M, et al. The edge-to-edge technique: a simplified method to correct mitral insufficiency. *Eur J Cardiothorac Surg.* 1998;13:240–245.
46. Alfieri O, Maisano F, De Bonis M, et al. The double-orifice technique in mitral valve repair: a simple solution for complex problems. *J Thorac Cardiovasc Surg.* 2001;122:674–681.
47. Maisano F, Schreuder JJ, Oppizzi M, et al. The double-orifice technique as a standardized approach to treat mitral regurgitation due to severe myxomatous disease: surgical technique. *Eur J Cardiothorac Surg.* 2000;17:201–205.
48. Lorusso R, Borghetti V, Totaro P, et al. The double-orifice technique for mitral valve reconstruction: predictors of postoperative outcome. *Eur J Cardiothorac Surg.* 2001;20:583–589.
49. Agricola E, Maisano F, Oppizzi M, et al. Mitral valve reserve in double-orifice technique: an exercise echocardiographic study. *J Heart Valve Dis.* 2002;11:637–643.
50. Umana JP, Salehizadeh B, DeRose JJ Jr, et al. Bow-tie mitral valve repair: an adjuvant technique for ischemic mitral regurgitation. *Ann Thorac Surg.* 1998;66:1640–1646.
51. Totaro P, Tulumello E, Fellini P, et al. Mitral valve repair for isolated prolapse of the anterior leaflet: an 11-year follow-up. *Eur J Cardiothorac Surg.* 1999;15:119–126.
52. Kherani AR, Cheema FH, Casher J, et al. Edge-to-edge mitral valve repair: the Columbia Presbyterian experience. *Ann Thorac Surg.* 2004;78:73–76.

53. Kinnaird TD, Munt BI, Ignaszewski AP, Abel JG, Thompson RC. Edge-to-edge repair for functional mitral regurgitation: an echocardiographic study of the hemodynamic consequences. *J Heart Valve Dis.* 2003;12:280–286.
54. Kallner G, van der Linden J, Hadjinikolaou L, Lindblom D. Transaortic approach for the Alfieri stitch. *Ann Thorac Surg.* 2001;71:378–379.
55. Gatti G, Cardu G, Trane R, Pugliese P. The edge-to-edge technique as a trick to rescue an imperfect mitral valve repair. *Eur J Cardiothorac Surg.* 2002;22:817–820.
56. Chauvaud S, Jebara V, Chachques JC, et al. Valve extension with glutaraldehyde-preserved autologous pericardium. Results in mitral valve repair. *J Thorac Cardiovasc Surg.* 1991;102:171–177.
57. Ng CK, Nesser J, Punzengruber C, et al. Valvuloplasty with glutaraldehyde-treated autologous pericardium in patients with complex mitral valve pathology. *Ann Thorac Surg.* 2001;71:78–85.
58. van der Lee C, Kofflard MJ, van Herwerden LA, Vletter WB, ten Cate FJ. Sustained improvement after combined anterior mitral leaflet extension and myectomy in hypertrophic obstructive cardiomyopathy. *Circulation.* 2003;108:2088–2092.
59. Hisatomi K, Isomura T, Hirano A, et al. Long-term follow-up results after reconstruction of the mitral valve by leaflet advancement. *Ann Thorac Surg.* 1992;54:271–275.
60. Sauvage LR, Wood SJ. Technique for correction of mitral insufficiency by leaflet advancement. *J Thorac Cardiovasc Surg.* 1964;49:752.
61. Sauvage LR, Wood SJ, Berger KE, Campbell AA. Autologous pericardium for leaflet advancement. *J Thorac Cardiovasc Surg.* 1966;52:849–854.
62. Chauvaud S, Jebara V, Chachques JC, et al. Valve extension with glutaraldehyde-preserved autologous pericardium. Results in mitral valve repair. *J Thorac Cardiovasc Surg.* 1991;102:171–177.
63. Kincaid EH, Riley RD, Hines MH, Hammon JW, Kon ND. Anterior leaflet augmentation for ischemic mitral regurgitation. *Ann Thorac Surg.* 2004;78:564–568.

Complications and Assessing the Quality of Repair

12

INTRAOPERATIVE ASSESSMENT OF VALVE COMPETENCE

The simplest and most reliable method to assess valve competence is to rapidly and forcibly inject saline through the valve to fill and distend the left ventricle and aortic root. This can be done with a 20 Fr. red rubber catheter attached to a bulb syringe. The catheter is inserted through the valve and rapidly withdrawn after the injection. Multiple injections may be necessary to ensure adequate ventricular distension to pull the leaflets down below the annular plane; a competent valve may leak if ventricular filling is not adequate to allow valvular coaptation. When evaluating the valve leaflets the entire line of closure should be parallel to the mural part of the annulus (1). Approximately 0.5 cm or more of tissue apposition along the entire line of closure is important. Focal areas of inadequate apposition should be evaluated closely as they may be sites of potential early failure (Figs. 12.1–12.5). Any residual leaflet prolapse, even in the absence of a leak, should be addressed to prevent early failure.

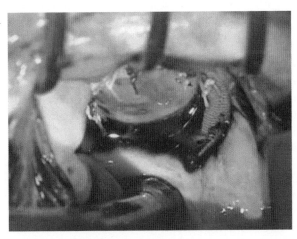

Figure 12.1   Testing the valve after ring placement. (Clip 5, Case 2)

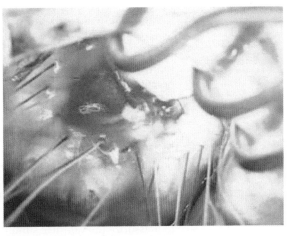

Figure 12.2   Intraoperative evaluation of a posterior leaflet cleft after a posterior sliding plasty. (Clip 6, Case 1)

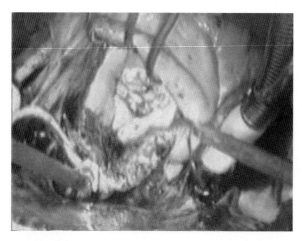

Figure 12.3   Testing after ring placement. (Clip 6, Case 5)

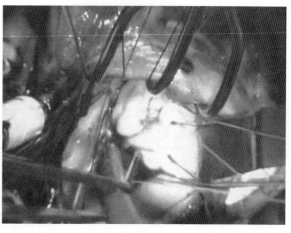

Figure 12.4   Testing the valve after medial commissuro-plasty. (Clip 7, Case 4)

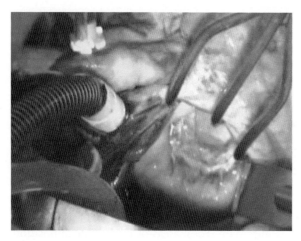

Figure 12.5   Final test after band placement. (Clip 11, Case 1)

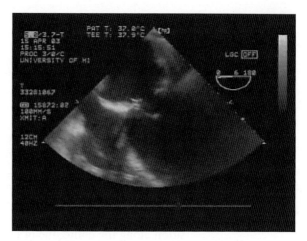

Figure 12.6   Postoperative echocardiogram showing reduced annular diameter. (Clip 6, Case 2)

Once the heart is beating and the patient has been weaned from cardiopulmonary bypass, the valve should be evaluated using transesophageal echocardiography as described in Chapter 4. Intraoperative echocardiography identified early failures (8%) that were immediately addressed (2). Any leak more than trace or 1+ should be evaluated closely because the long-term rate of failure will be higher with 2+ or more regurgitation (3). As a rule-of-thumb, any degree of regurgitation noted intraoperatively will increase by 1 in the awake patient. If regurgitation is noted the systolic blood pressure should be raised with vasoconstrictor agents to between 150 and 160 mmHg to assure the degree of regurgitation remains unchanged (Figs. 12.6–12.8).

Another method of assessment is to infuse blood into the aortic root, allowing the heart to beat with the aortic cross-clamp in place to assess dynamic function (Fig. 12.9). This can be used before repair to assess the site of leak and after repair to assess the adequacy of repair (4). Alternatively, an additional cannula can be placed through the ventricular apex to pressurize the ventricle simultaneous with aortic root perfusion (Fig. 12.10) (5). In most scenarios these techniques are unnecessary and more useful in the assessment of excessive regurgitation noted on echocardiography after competency was noted with saline infusion through the valve.

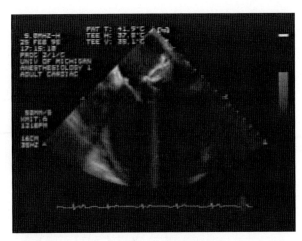

Figure 12.7 Postoperative echocardiogram dilated cardiomyopathy. (Clip 7, Case 5)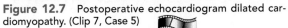

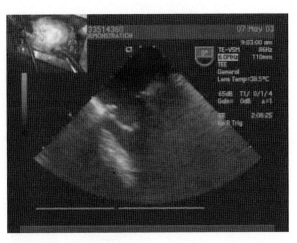

Figure 12.8 Postoperative echocardiogram. (Clip 9, Case 4)

If combined aortic and mitral procedures are performed, the mitral repair should be completed and tested before opening the aorta. If the aorta must be opened prior to repair (e.g., to administer cardioplegia in the presence of aortic insufficiency) the aorta can be clamped below the aortotomy. Alternatively, a foley catheter can be passed through the annulus, the balloon inflated, and the catheter wedged in the outflow tract; fluid for distension can then be infused through the lumen of the catheter to distend the ventricle and test the valve (6) (Fig. 12.11).

SYSTOLIC ANTERIOR MOTION (SAM)

Systolic anterior motion (SAM) occurs when the anterior leaflet is caught in the stream of ejecting blood and pulled anteriorly toward the septum rather than closing by moving posteriorly, causing left ventricular outflow tract obstruction and mitral regurgitation (Fig. 12.12).

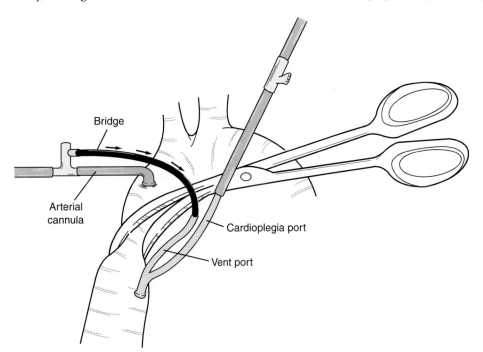

Figure 12.9 Aortic root perfusion for assessment of the mitral valve in the beating heart. (From Marshall Jr. WG. Technique for visualization of the functioning mitral valve. *Ann Thorac Surg.* 1990;49:1013.)

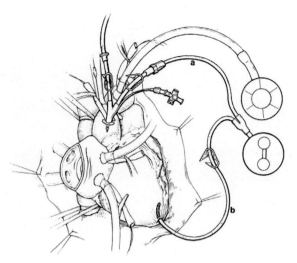

Figure 12.10 Setup for controlled root and ventricular perfusion to assess the mitral valve in the beating heart. (From Sundt 3rd TM, Khaghani A, Yacoub MH. Alternative technique for assessment and repair of the mitral valve. *Ann Thorac Surg.* 1996;61:1552–1554.)

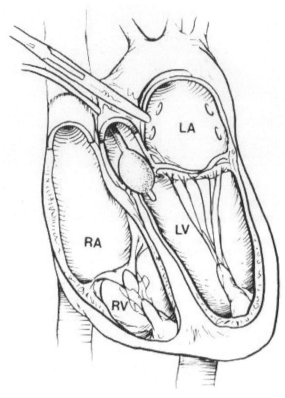

Figure 12.11 Occlusion of the left ventricular outflow tract with a foley catheter to test the mitral repair with an open aorta. (From Ferguson Jr. TB, Wechsler AS. Testing of mitral valve competence following combined mitral valve repair and aortic valve replacement. *Ann Thorac Surg.* 1985;40,631–633.)

Originally reported to occur in between 4.5% and 10% of patients (7), the incidence is much lower with newer repair techniques (8,9). SAM is more common in patients with smaller ventricles and taller posterior leaflets (10). SAM was noted when the ratio of the length of the anterior to the posterior leaflet was small (0.99 with SAM, 1.95 without SAM) (11). The general consensus is that SAM is caused by anterior displacement of the site of coaptation of the leaflets secondary to excessive height or redundant tissue in the posterior leaflet (12,13,14). Anterior displacement was attributed to annular plication of the annulus after extensive (>3 cm) quadrangular resection and leaflet prolapse (15). This can be avoided by alternative posterior leaflet techniques, such as posterior leaflet sliding plasty (see Chapter 9), when large portions of the posterior leaflet are resected and avoiding an annuloplasty ring that is too small (10). SAM has been reported to be associated with the use of a rigid annuloplasty ring (15), but can occur with a flexible ring (16) or in the absence of a ring (17).

SAM is most commonly noted intraoperatively, and is usually associated with hypotension, hypovolemia, a small ventricular cavity, ventricular hypertrophy, and a hyperdynamic

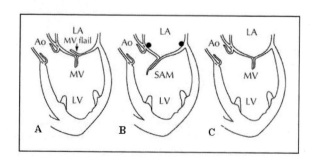

Figure 12.12 Systolic anterior motion (SAM); **A:** Before repair; **B:** SAM after repair; **C:** elimination of SAM after rerepair. (From Lee KS, Stewart WJ, Lever HM, Underwood PL, Cosgrove DM. Mechanism of outflow obstruction following failed valve repair: anterior displacement of leaflet coaptation. *Circulation.* 1993;88 (Suppl II):II-24-9.)

state induced by catecholamine use. In most cases, it will resolve with withdrawal of inotropic stimuli, volume loading, slowing heart rate to increase ventricular filling, and increasing afterload to reduce ventricular emptying. Raney et al. used the "Pomeroy Procedure" or anterior leaflet shortening (Chapter 8) described above to correct SAM in one patient (18). If persistent after above measures an alternative to repair revision is transaortic septal myectomy, used in two patients by Rescigno et al. (19) and five patients by Civelek et al. (20).

HEMOLYTIC ANEMIA

Hemolytic anemia secondary to the repair usually presents within the first few months, and has been attributed to a high velocity jet directed at the cloth-covered annuloplasty ring (21). However, it can be associated with high shear stress due to the regurgitant jet (22,23). It can occur in the presence of mild regurgitation (24). The diagnosis of hemolytic anemia is suggested by increased serum haptoglobin, elevation of serum lactate dehydrogenase (LDH), and schistocytosis. This may improve over time if the ring heals in (though the regurgitant jet may prevent this) (25). Beta-blockers have been used to reduce the velocity of the regurgitant jet. Reoperation is often necessary and re-repair is possible.

STENOSIS

Early stenosis is unusual and late stenosis is rare. Reviewing 478 patients with regurgitation secondary to nonrheumatic etiology repaired with various rings and bands, 4 patients developed late stenosis secondary to pannus overgrowth on the annuloplasty ring, extending onto the leaflets (26). This occurred in a subgroup of 138 patients repaired with a Duran ring.

MISCELLANEOUS RESULTS

A number of groups have reported long-term results that have been summarized in Table 12.1. Valve repair has also been performed with good success in the presence of endocarditis (27,28). Causes of reoperation were discussed for 49 patients by Cerfolio et al. Reasons for reoperation included recurrent severe regurgitation (70%), hemolytic anemia (14%), mixed regurgitation and stenosis (14%), and mitral stenosis (2%). In 65% the initial repairs were intact. Regurgitation was due to fibrosis and calcification, ruptured chordae, or leaflet perforations. Causes of regurgitation when the repair had failed included dehiscence of commissural repairs or the ring annuloplasty, or breakdown of chordal or leaflet repair. Operative mortality for the second procedure was 4%; most were replaced but 16% were re-repaired (29). Gillinov et al. reviewed 86 reoperations in 81 patients. They categorized failures as procedure related, valve related, or of unknown cause. Fifty of the failures (58%) were procedure related and included suture dehiscence, 21; rupture of previously shortened chordae, 19; or incomplete correction, 10. Valve-related failures (33, 38%) included progressive disease, 27; endocarditis, 5; or leaflet retraction, 1. In the remaining failures (3, 3%) no cause could be identified. Seventy percent of failures were procedure related with valves affected by degenerative disease; whereas most failures with rheumatic disease valves were related to progression of disease. Re-repair was performed in 21%. They concluded that chordal shortening should not be used (30).

WHEN TO GIVE UP

One lasting concern for surgeons is the effect of immediate failure, requiring subsequent replacement on operative modality. Northrup et al. investigated this, comparing morbidity and mortality among patients who underwent repair with those whose repair failed and required replacement during the same operation (31). No increase in morbidity or mortality was conferred by the failed attempt despite longer cross clamp, perfusion, and operative times.

TABLE 12.1
RESULTS OF MITRAL VALVE REPAIR

Author	Date of Publication	Number of Patients (Hospital Survivors)	Freedom from Reoperation Years/%	Note
Fernandez (32)	1992	313	5y/90%, 8y/80%* 5y/80%, 10y/72%**	Pure MR or MS* Mixed MS/MR** Less durability with rheumatic etiology and greater with ischemic etiology
Thourani (33)	2003	625	5y/94%, 10y/78%	+ 10 years freedom from reoperation with replacement was 66%
Fucci (34)	1995	299	7y/86%	At 7 years freedom from reoperation for anterior triangular resection was 61%; anterior chordal shortening, 56%; ischemic etiology, 51%
Gillinov (35,36)	1998	1072	10y/93%	Degenerative disease only Durability reduced with chordal shortening, annuloplasty alone, leaflet resection without annuloplasty For posterior quadrangular resection with annuloplasty 98% (36)

The quality of the repair at the time of surgery is the best guide for indicator of long-term success or failure. The greater the amount of residual mitral regurgitation, the greater the risk of recurrence. The disease process also dictates failure rates, rheumatic higher for others. The complexity of the repair may contribute to long-term failures. Finally, the amount of experience the surgeon has with repair will impact long-term results. The threshold for abandoning the repair and replacing the valve is an individual decision and should be based on all of these contributing factors.

FOLLOW-UP

An echocardiogram to assess the repair is recommended prior to hospital discharge. Technical failures will occur early and are easiest to address in the early postoperative period. Anticoagulation is surgeon dependent with no agreed upon strategies. Some surgeons treat only with aspirin, others use warfarin for 2 to 3 months until the ring or band becomes incorporated. An alternative might be a selective strategy, treating simple annuloplasty with aspirin and using warfarin for more complex repairs. Hypertension control is important. Many of these patients are on afterload-reducing medications, which should be continued in the early postoperative period. Activities that increase blood pressure, such as weightlifting, should be restricted until healing is complete.

REFERENCES

1. Carpentier A. Cardiac valve surgery: the "French Correction." *J Thorac Cardiovasc Surg.* 1986;86:323.
2. Marwick TH, Stewart WJ, Currie PJ, Cosgrove DM. Mechanisms of failure of mitral valve repair: an echocardiographic study. *Am Heart J.* 1991;122:149–156.
3. Fix J, Isada L, Cosgrove DM, et al. Do patients with less than "echo-perfect" results from mitral valve repair by intraoperative echocardiography have a different outcome? *Circulation.* 1993;88:39.
4. Marshall Jr. WG. Technique for visualization of the functioning mitral valve. *Ann Thorac Surg.* 1990;49:1013.
5. Sundt TM 3rd, Khaghani A, Yacoub MH. Alternative technique for assessment and repair of the mitral valve. *Ann Thorac Surg.* 1996;61:1552–1554.
6. Ferguson Jr. TB, Wechsler AS. Testing of mitral valve competence following combined mitral valve repair and aortic valve replacement. *Ann Thorac Surg.* 1985;40:631–633.
7. Kreindel MS, Schiavone WA, Lever HM, Cosgrove DM. Systolic anterior motion of the mitral valve after Carpentier ring valvuloplasty for mitral valve prolapse. *Am J Cardiol.* 1986;57:408.
8. Jebara VA, Mihaileanu S, Acar C, et al. Left ventricular outflow obstruction after mitral valve repair: results of the sliding leaflet technique. *Circulation.* 1993;88 (Part 2):30.
9. Perier P, Clausnizer B, Mistarz K. Carpentier "sliding leaflet" technique for repair of the mitral valve: early results. *Ann Thorac Surg.* 1994;57:383.
10. Sanders JH Jr, Scott ML. Pitfalls in surgical decision-making during mitral valve repair. *Curr Opin Cardiol.* 2001;16:140–145.
11. Maslow AD, Regan MM, Haering JM, Johnson RG, Levine RA. Echocardiographic predictors of left ventricular outflow tract obstruction and systolic anterior motion of the mitral valve after mitral valve reconstruction for myxomatous valve disease. *J Am Coll Cardiol.* 1999;34:2096–2104.
12. He S, Hopmeyer J, Lefebvre XP, et al. Importance of leaflet elongation in causing systolic anterior motion of the mitral valve. *J Heart Valve Dis.* 1997;6:149–159.
13. Lee KS, Stewart WJ, Lever HM, Underwood PL, Cosgrove DM. Mechanism of outflow obstruction following failed valve repair: anterior displacement of leaflet coaptation. *Circulation.* 1993;88 (Suppl II): II-24-9.
14. Mihaileanu S, Marino JP, Chauvaud S, et al. Left ventricular outflow obstruction after mitral repair (Carpentier's technique): proposed mechanism of disease. *Circulation.* 1988;78 (Suppl I):78–84.
15. Grossi EA, Galloway AC, Parish MA, et al. Experience with twenty-eight cases of systolic motion after mitral valve construction by Carpentier technique. *J Thorac Cardiovasc Surg.* 1992;103:466–470.
16. Lopez JA, Schnee M, Gaos CM, Wilansky S. Left ventricular outflow tract obstruction and hemolytic anemia after mitral valve repair with a Duran ring. *Ann Thorac Surg.* 1994;58:876–867.
17. Kupferschmid JP, Carr T, Connelly GP, Shemin RJ. Systolic anterior motion of the mitral valve after valve repair without an annular ring. *Ann Thorac Surg.* 1994;57:484–486.
18. Raney AA, Shah PM, Joyo CI. The "Pomeroy procedure": a new method to correct post-mitral valve repair systolic anterior motion. *J Heart Valve Dis.* 2001;10:307–311.
19. Rescigno G, Matteucci MLS, Iacovoni A, et al. Systolic anterior motion after mitral valve repair: myectomy as an alternative solution. *J Thorac Cardiovasc Surg.* 2003;126:1196–1197.
20. Civelek A, Szalay Z, Roth M, et al. Post-mitral valve repair systolic anterior motion produced by non-obstructive septal bulge. *Eur J Cardiothorac Surg.* 2003;24:857–861.
21. Wilson JH, Rath R, Glaser R, Panke T. Severe hemolysis after incomplete mitral valve repair. *Ann Thorac Surg.* 1990;50:136–137.
22. Garcia MJ, Vandervoort P, Stewart WJ, et al. Mechanisms of hemolysis with mitral prosthetic regurgitation. Study using transesophageal echocardiography and fluid dynamic simulation. *J Am Coll Cardiol.* 1996;27:399–406.
23. Yeo TC, Freeman WK, Schaff HV, Orszulak TA. Mechanisms of hemolysis after mitral valve repair: assessment by serial echocardiography. *J Am Coll Cardiol.* 1998;32:717–723.
24. Cerfolio RJ, Orszulak TA, Daly RC, Schaff HV. Reoperation for hemolytic anaemia complicating mitral valve repair. *Eur J Cardiothorac Surg.* 1997;11:479–484.
25. Inoue M, Kaku B, Kanaya H, et al. Reduction of hemolysis without reoperation following mitral valve repair. *Circ J.* 2003;67:799–801.
26. Ibrahim MF, David TE. Mitral stenosis after mitral valve repair for non-rheumatic mitral regurgitation. *Ann Thorac Surg.* 2002;73:34–36.
27. Dreyfus G, Serraf A, Jebara VA, et al. Valve repair in acute endocarditis. *Ann Thorac Surg.* 1990;49:706–711.
28. Hendren WG, Morris AS, Rosenkranz ER, et al. Mitral valve repair for bacterial endocarditis. *J Thorac Cardiovasc Surg.* 1992;103:124–128.
29. Cerfolio RJ, Orzulak TA, Pluth JR, Harmsen WS, Schaff HV. Reoperation after valve repair for mitral regurgitation: early and intermediate results. *J Thorac Cardiovasc Surg.* 1996;111:1177–1183.
30. Gillinov AM, Cosgrove DM, Lytle BW, et al. Reoperation for failure of mitral valve repair. *J Thorac Cardiovasc Surg.* 1997;113:467–473.
31. Northrup 3rd WF, DuBois KA, Kshettry VR. Morbidity and mortality of a failed attempt at mitral valve repair converted to replacement at the same operation. *J Heart Valve Dis.* 2003;12:700–706.
32. Fernandez J, Joyce DH, Hirschfeld K, et al. Factors affecting mitral valve reoperation in 317 survivors after mitral valve reconstruction. *Ann Thorac Surg.* 1992;54:440–447.
33. Thourani VH, Weintraub WS, Guyton RA, et al. Outcomes and long-term survival for patients undergoing mitral valve repair versus replacement: effect of age and concomitant coronary artery bypass grafting. *Circulation.* 2003;108:298–304.
34. Fucci C, Sandrelli L, Pardini A, et al. Improved results with mitral valve repair using new surgical techniques. *Eur J Cardiothorac Surg.* 1995;9:621–626.
35. Gillinov AM, Cosgrove DM, Blackstone EH, et al. Durability of mitral valve repair for degenerative disease. *J Thorac Cardiovasc Surg.* 1998;116:734–743.
36. Gillinov AM, Cosgrove DM. Mitral valve repair for degenerative disease. *J Heart Valve Dis.* 2002;11 Suppl 1:S15–20.

Index